PILATES
ANATOMY

General Disclaimer

The contents of this book are intended to provide useful information to the general public. All materials, including texts, graphics, and images, are for informational purposes only and are not a substitute for medical diagnosis, advice, or treatment for specific medical conditions. All readers should seek expert medical care and consult their own physicians before commencing any exercise program or for any general or specific health issues. The author and publishers do not recommend or endorse specific treatments, procedures, advice, or other information found in this book and specifically disclaim all responsibility for any and all liability, loss, or risk, personal or otherwise, which is incurred as a consequence, directly or indirectly, of the use or application of any of the material in this publication.

Thunder Bay Press
An imprint of the Baker & Taylor Publishing Group
10350 Barnes Canyon Road, San Diego, CA 92121
www.thunderbaybooks.com

Copyright © 2009 by Moseley Road Inc.

All notations of errors or omissions should be addressed to Thunder Bay Press, Editorial Department, at the above address. All other correspondence (author inquiries, permissions) concerning the content of this book should be addressed to Moseley Road, Inc., 129 Main Street, Irvington, NY 10533. www.moseleyroad.com.

ISBN-13: 978-1-60710-015-7
ISBN-10: 1-60710-015-0

Printed in Canada

1 2 3 4 5 13 12 11 10 09

PILATES
ANATOMY

A Comprehensive Guide

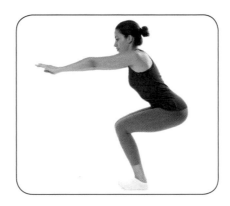

Dr. Abby Ellsworth

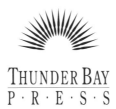

THUNDER BAY
P·R·E·S·S

San Diego, California

CONTENTS

INTRODUCTION

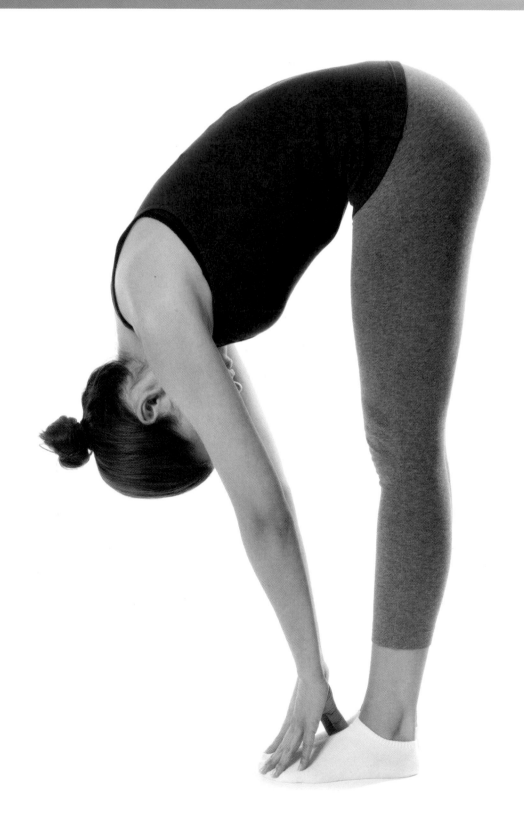

Since Joseph H. Pilates began developing his method of body conditioning nearly a century ago, Pilates has become one of the most popular ways to get fit and strong. Increasing numbers of people have come to embrace Pilates as an invigorating and fun way to not only get in shape, but to also discover things about the body that they didn't know before. Pilates offers endless possibilities with its scores of exercises based on six principles. As you look through this book, keep in mind that the exercises featured here are only an introduction to Pilates. Thousands of exercises exist and infinite variations are available, making it easy to craft a program aligned with each individual's needs. Yet, the six principles must always be preserved.

Pilates Anatomy highlights some of the main exercises that are considered the foundation of "classical" Pilates training. This foundation will provide you with a base from which to build, allowing you to take your Pilates experience as far as you wish.

You can use this book in several ways. As a novice, you will most likely want to focus on the basic principles before you move along to more difficult exercises. If you already have a good knowledge of Pilates, you'll find a number of exercises to add to your routine. Step-by-step photos and anatomical illustrations guide you through the exercise movements, with the muscles active in each exercise highlighted. There are also handy tips that note each exercise's focus to better allow you to target certain areas of your body. The exercises are grouped into three sections—Beginner, Intermediate, and Advanced—and each section features sample workout sequences so that you can test your skills as you progress.

THE PILATES METHOD

The Pilates method aims to strengthen your core, or "center," lengthen the spine, build muscle tone, and increase body awareness. Following the six principles below will help you gain all of these benefits while maintaining safety.

❶ CONTROL

Joseph Pilates originally called his method of exercise Contrology. The principle of control is the main focus of his exercise system. Control is important in everything we do—especially on the Pilates mat. It is crucial at the beginning (initiation) and at the end of each movement, because mat exercises are based on the resistance provided by your body's weight and gravity.

As you work out, the control of your muscles, positions, and speed gives you results and keeps you safe. This rule not only applies to the routines themselves, but also to the transitions between exercises. By mastering the principle of control, you will train your muscles to maintain a strong and lengthened state throughout the entire movement, reducing muscle bulk in the process. While focusing on control, you are also encouraging your body to recruit smaller "helper" muscles, known as synergists, which aid the muscles of the body in working together. These synergists are the key to developing coordination and balance through movement.

❷ BREATH

Have you ever caught yourself holding your breath while lifting something heavy or carrying out a difficult task? Holding your breath builds pressure in the muscles and spinal cord and changes heart rhythm and blood pressure. Deep, consistent breathing is essential to a flowing movement, proper muscle balance, and overall health.

Most people do not know how to breathe correctly, and consequently use about half of their available lung capacity. Shallow breathing is the result of several outside factors, including stress, smoking, and a sedentary lifestyle. Learning how to breathe correctly is crucial for healthy living and an increased lung capacity.

Controlled breathing is a core aspect of Pilates, and this emphasis sets it apart from other exercise forms. If you are just beginning and feel confused about when to breathe and what type of breath to use, remember this general rule of thumb: when in doubt, exhale during the most difficult part of the exercise.

There are three main types of breathing utilized in Pilates, each with its own purpose and benefits. As you become more familiar with the types of breathing and the exercises, your body will help you naturally select the one that is appropriate for the movement, so don't worry if you feel overwhelmed at first and are not sure which way to breathe.

THE ACCORDION OR BILLOWS BREATHING

Place your hands on either side of your rib cage. Take a deep breath in and let the space between your hands expand to the sides (creating a big gap in the middle). Then breathe out (exhale), slowly allowing the rib cage to decrease in size and letting your hands come together. Allow all of the air to leave your lungs, and feel your abdominal muscles activate to assist. Repeat, practicing the lateral (sideways) expansion of the rib cage. This lateral expansion allows the ribs to remain stable on the spine and keeps the torso balanced.

PERCUSSIVE BREATHING

The percussive breathing method is smooth and deep on the inhale and percussive (resisted) on the exhale. You should be able to feel the abdominals forcing the air out of your lungs on the exhale, and you can use a *shh, shh* sound with the breath out. This breathing is typically used for the Hundred exercise.

EVEN BREATHING

This technique allows breathing without displacing any part of your body. The inhale and exhale occur without a lot of movement in the rib cage or stomach.

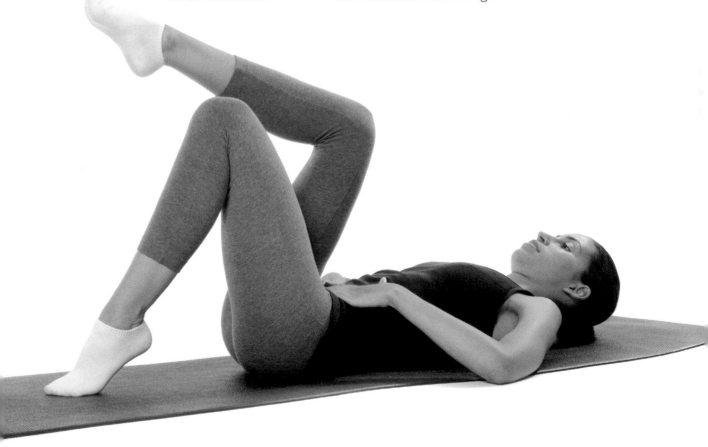

THE PILATES METHOD

PRINCIPLES

❸ FLOW OF MOVEMENT

The essence of Pilates exercises is to allow your body to move freely with control and precision, encouraging flexibility in the joints and muscles and teaching the body to move and elongate with even rhythm. Balanced movement that flows smoothly integrates the nervous system, muscles, and joints and trains the body to move in an even and dynamic fashion.

❹ PRECISION

Precision combines control with the spatial awareness of movement. The beginning and end of each movement is paramount. All exercises require precise positioning of the body throughout the movement. This principle is one of the most important in the entire Pilates system—precision will help you get the most from your workout and protect you from injury.

❺ CENTERING

Pulling your navel toward your spine is a great way to bring your deep abdominal muscles into action. These deep abdominal muscles are the keys to finding your center and helping to ensure proper stability with each exercise. Once your center is activated, you can move dynamically through each movement with control and precision.

❻ STABILITY

The majority of the Pilates mat exercises focus on torso stability. Stability is maintained by restricting or preventing movement in one part of the body while another part is moving. In order to achieve stability, you must activate your core to prevent movement through the spine. This allows your arms and legs to move with precision while creating a stable surface on which the rest of the body can move freely.

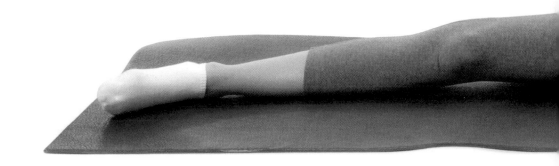

CONTINUED

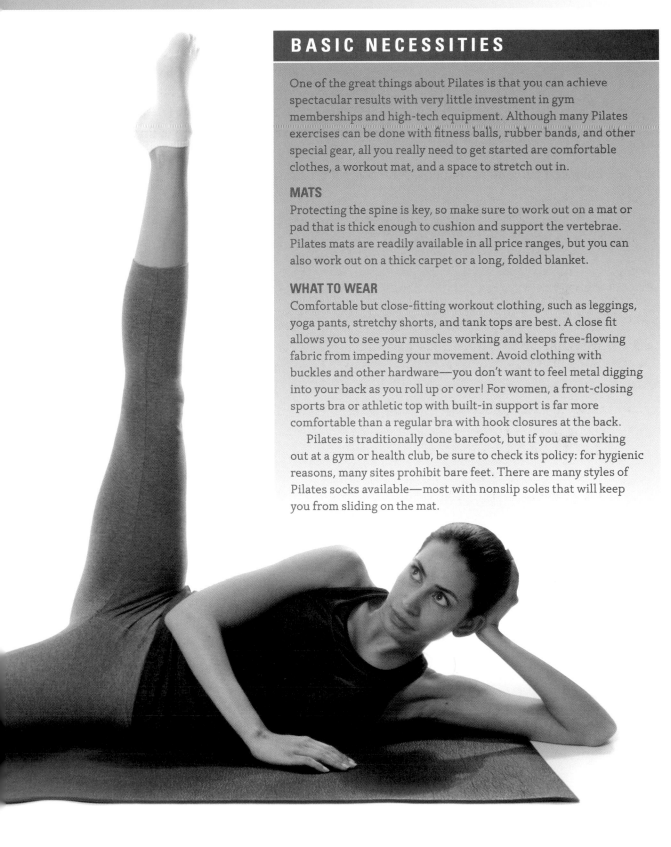

BASIC NECESSITIES

One of the great things about Pilates is that you can achieve spectacular results with very little investment in gym memberships and high-tech equipment. Although many Pilates exercises can be done with fitness balls, rubber bands, and other special gear, all you really need to get started are comfortable clothes, a workout mat, and a space to stretch out in.

MATS

Protecting the spine is key, so make sure to work out on a mat or pad that is thick enough to cushion and support the vertebrae. Pilates mats are readily available in all price ranges, but you can also work out on a thick carpet or a long, folded blanket.

WHAT TO WEAR

Comfortable but close-fitting workout clothing, such as leggings, yoga pants, stretchy shorts, and tank tops are best. A close fit allows you to see your muscles working and keeps free-flowing fabric from impeding your movement. Avoid clothing with buckles and other hardware—you don't want to feel metal digging into your back as you roll up or over! For women, a front-closing sports bra or athletic top with built-in support is far more comfortable than a regular bra with hook closures at the back.

Pilates is traditionally done barefoot, but if you are working out at a gym or health club, be sure to check its policy: for hygienic reasons, many sites prohibit bare feet. There are many styles of Pilates socks available—most with nonslip soles that will keep you from sliding on the mat.

PILATES BASICS

BASICS

In addition to the six core principles of Pilates, there are several basics and body positions that you'll return to again and again. Take a few moments to learn this terminology so an unfamiliar phrase or pose doesn't detract from your valuable workout time. Much like the principles, these basics are helpful to keep in mind in all stages of your warm-up and exercise. Ensuring that your spine and abdomen are correctly engaged and that you begin and end each exercise in the proper position will set the stage for successful results.

SUPINE POSITION

The supine position requires that you lie on your back.

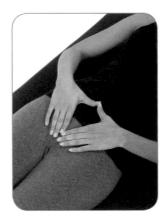

NEUTRAL SPINE

"Maintaining a neutral spine" means to keep the natural curves of the spine in the supine position. Pelvic neutral can be found by placing the hands in a triangle position over the pubic bone and hip bones.

LENGTHENING

Lengthening elongates the body's parts to create as much space and muscle length as possible.

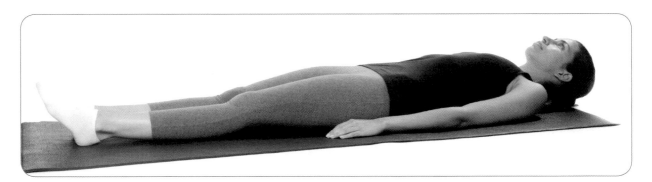

PRONE POSITION

The prone position requires that you lie on your stomach.

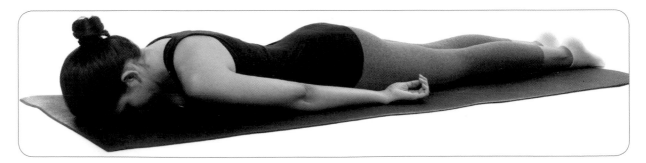

C CURVE

The "C" describes the shape of the back or spine after you scoop in your stomach. This position provides a stretch for the muscles surrounding your spine.

SCOOPING ABDOMINALS

Scooping in the abdominals works much like a drawstring pulled tightly around a pair of sweatpants. The scooping action brings in to play all four abdominals, which work to compress the abdominal wall and help support the back.

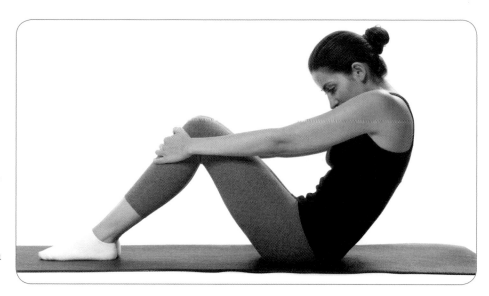

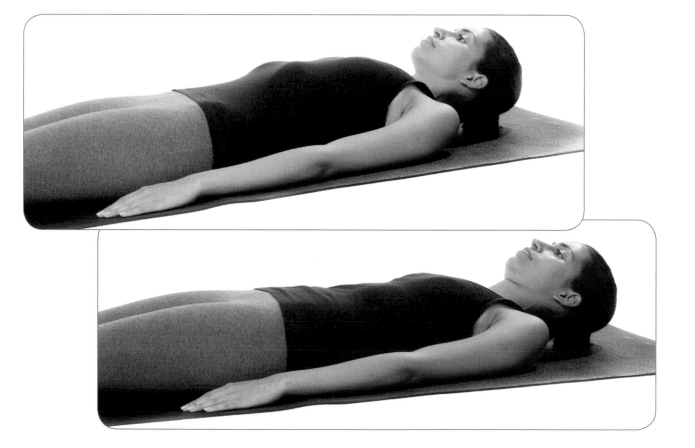

PILATES BASICS

BASICS

BALANCE POINT

The balance point is the point at which the body can balance on the pelvis while the feet are raised and the arms are either placed on the legs or in the air.

ARTICULATION

"Articulation" means to move one segment at a time and isolating the movement. The term most often refers to the spine and the vertebrae with an up or down motion.

STACKING THE SPINE

To stack the spine is to start with one part of the torso (either the shoulders or hips) and bend forward, articulating the spine one vertebra at a time until each vertebra is aligned one on top of another.

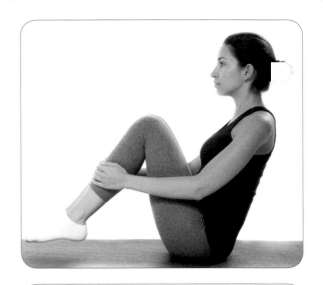

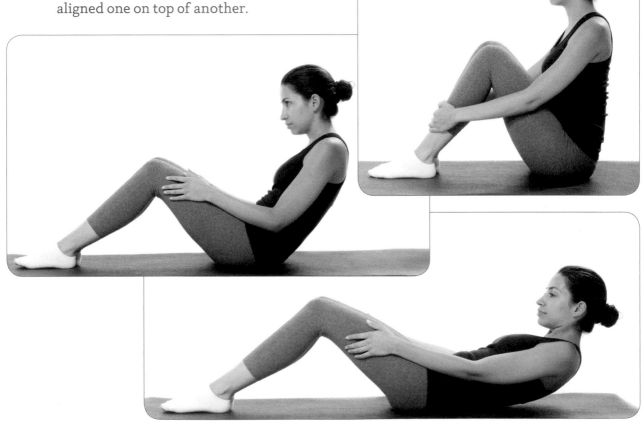

CONTINUED

PARALLEL POSITION VS. TURNOUT POSITION

The feet are aligned beside each other in the parallel position. In the turnout position, the heels touch while the toes are facing away from the body. The hips rotate outward to turn out the feet.

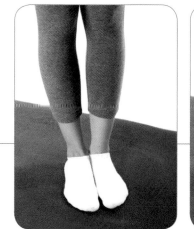
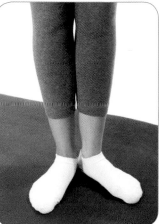

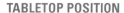

TABLETOP POSITION

While you lie in a supine position, the legs are raised, with a bend in the hips and the knees at a 90-degree angle, making the legs look like they are resting on the top of a table. The shins should be parallel to the ground and the feet should be flexed. The toes should be pointing straight up in the air.

OPPOSITION

In Pilates, "opposition" refers to the ability to create resistance in one's own body by either pushing against oneself or resisting a motion while moving through an exercise.

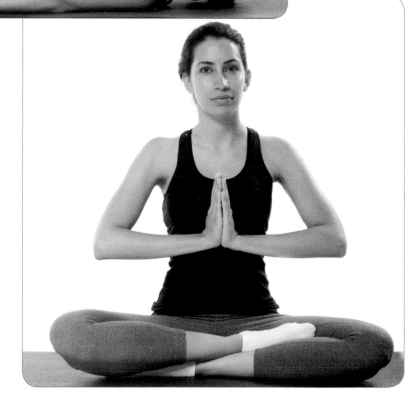

THE STRETCHES

Sufficient preparation is one of the most important things you can do to guarantee a safe, effective, and satisfying workout. For any exercise, warming up and stretching the muscles is crucial—in Pilates, warming up properly separates a mediocre workout from a great one. Because the exercises and movements in this book require you to engage very specific muscles, often in quick succession and for extended periods of time, you'll want your entire body to be as ready and limber as possible. Beginning with these stretches is a fantastic way to learn and reinforce the core principles of Pilates: control, breath, flow of movement, precision, centering, and stability. As you work on each muscle and movement in your warm-up, try to practice the same focus, awareness, and economy of movement that you'll maintain throughout the exercises in this book. Before long you'll start to discover exciting parallels and connections between the exercises and your muscles—and you'll be well on your way to a fitter, more flexible body.

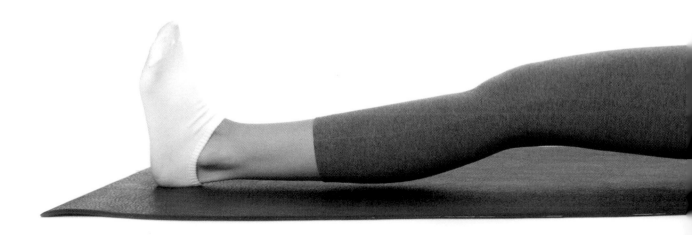

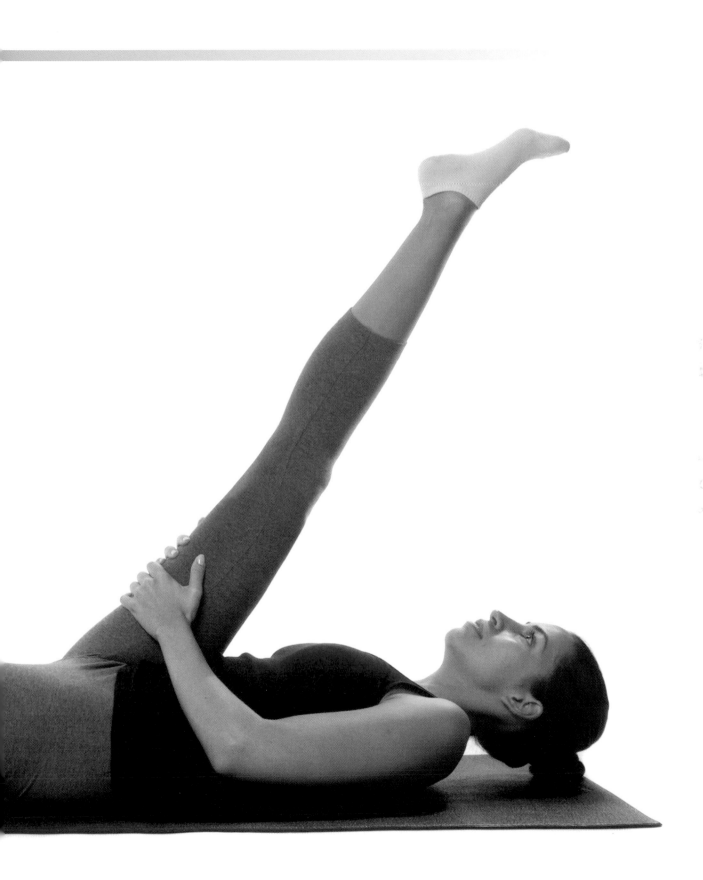

HAMSTRING STRETCH

STRETCHES

This simple but effective stretch is important in preparing the muscles of the legs for many of the exercises in this book. Take care not to overexert the biceps femoris, semitendinosus, and semimembranosus muscles—better known as the "hamstrings." Slow, deliberate stretching is best.

DO IT RIGHT

LOOK FOR
• Your lower back to remain on the floor.

AVOID
• Pulling your stretched leg so far that your other leg lifts off the mat.

❶ Lying flat on your back, raise one leg while supporting the back of your knee with your hand.

❷ Slowly straighten the knee until you feel the stretch in the back of your thigh.

latissimus dorsi

gluteus medius*

gluteus maximus

vastus lateralis

semitendinosus

biceps femoris

semimembranosus

ANNOTATION KEY
**Bold text indicates
active muscles**
Gray text indicates
stabilizing muscles
* indicates deep muscles

BEST FOR

• biceps femoris
• semitendinosus
• semimembranosus
• gluteus maximus

❸ Hold for fifteen seconds and then repeat sequence three times on each leg.

ITB STRETCH

BEST FOR

- iliotibial band
- biceps femoris
- gluteus maximus
- vastus lateralis

1. Standing, cross your left leg in front of your right.

2. Bend at the waist while keeping both knees straight, reaching your hands toward the floor.

3. Hold for fifteen seconds and repeat sequence three times on each leg.

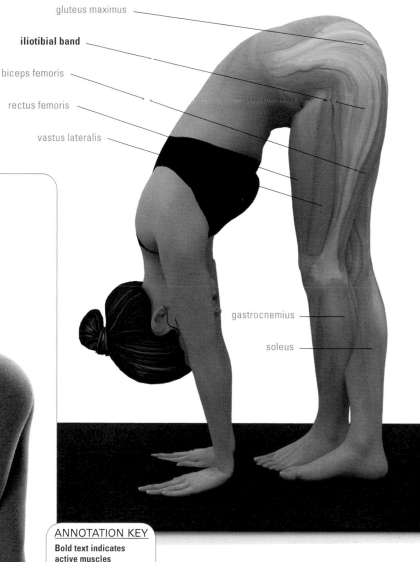

gluteus maximus

iliotibial band

biceps femoris

rectus femoris

vastus lateralis

gastrocnemius

soleus

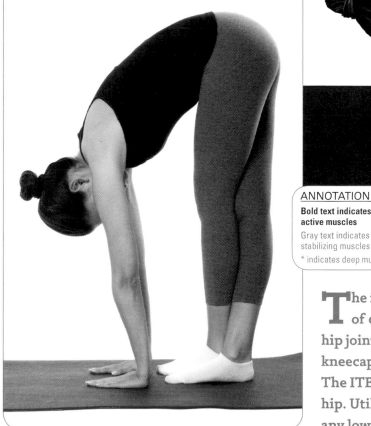

ANNOTATION KEY
Bold text indicates active muscles
Gray text indicates stabilizing muscles
* indicates deep muscles

The iliotibial band, or ITB, is a thick band of connective tissue that crosses the hip joint and extends down to insert on the kneecap, tibia, and biceps femoris tendon. The ITB stabilizes the knee and abducts the hip. Utilize this stretch before attempting any lower-body positions or exercises.

HIP FLEXOR STRETCH

STRETCHES

Improving hip flexibility is a cornerstone of any Pilates program. Performing this stretch before going on to other exercises will ensure that the hips are limber.

DO IT RIGHT

LOOK FOR
• Your head to face forward and your back to remain straight.

AVOID
• Pushing your front knee in past your ankle. The angle that your calf makes with the mat should not exceed 90 degrees.

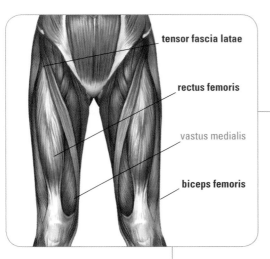

tensor fascia latae

rectus femoris

vastus medialis

biceps femoris

ANNOTATION KEY

Bold text indicates active muscles

Gray text indicates stabilizing muscles

* indicates deep muscles

❶ Kneeling, bring one leg forward, with your foot in front of your knee.

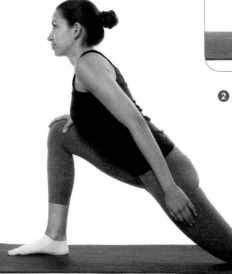

❷ Slowly lean forward and push your pelvis down until you feel a stretch in the front of your hip. Hold for fifteen seconds. Repeat sequence three times on each leg.

BEST FOR

• rectus femoris
• vastus medialis
• biceps femoris
• tensor fasciae latae

QUADRICEPS STRETCH

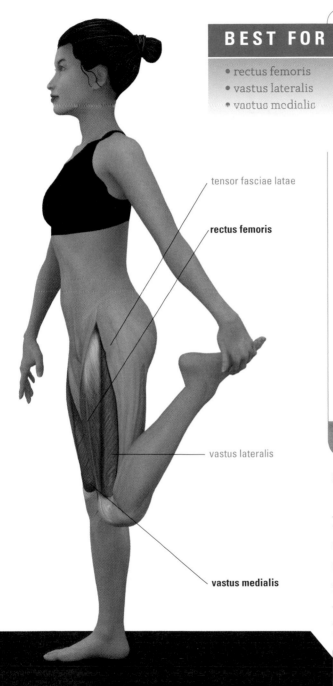

tensor fasciae latae

rectus femoris

vastus lateralis

vastus medialis

BEST FOR

- rectus femoris
- vastus lateralis
- vastus medialis

❶ Standing, pull your heel toward your buttocks with your hand until you feel a stretch in the front of your thigh. Keep both knees together and aligned.

❷ Hold for fifteen seconds. Repeat sequence three times on each leg.

The quadriceps, a group of four muscles (the vastus medialis, intermedius, and lateralis, along with the rectus femoris) that sit on the front aspect of the thigh, must be stretched in order to achieve full length and flexibility in the legs. Standing straight and tall without leaning and rocking will also help improve balance.

DO IT RIGHT

LOOK FOR
- Both knees to remain pressed together.

AVOID
- Leaning forward with your chest.

ANNOTATION KEY
Bold text indicates active muscles
Gray text indicates stabilizing muscles
* indicates deep muscles

RUNNER'S STRETCH

STRETCHES

Runners and athletes rely on this stretch every day, and it's useful for Pilates as well. For full-leg flexibility, don't forget this move.

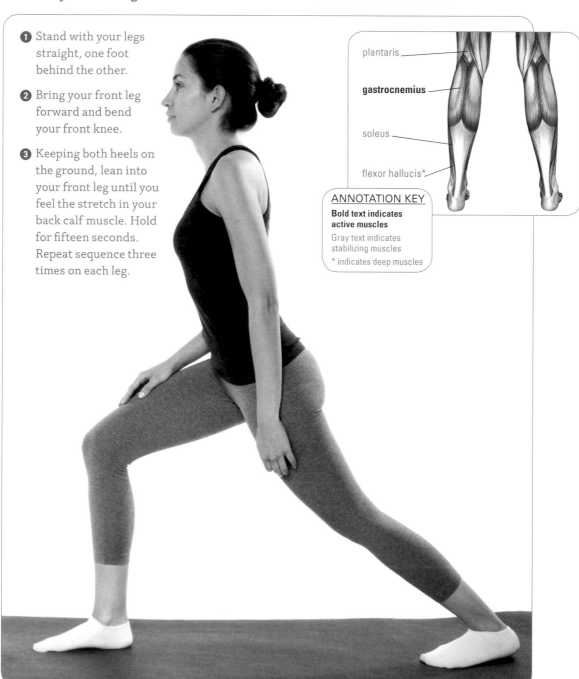

1. Stand with your legs straight, one foot behind the other.

2. Bring your front leg forward and bend your front knee.

3. Keeping both heels on the ground, lean into your front leg until you feel the stretch in your back calf muscle. Hold for fifteen seconds. Repeat sequence three times on each leg.

plantaris

gastrocnemius

soleus

flexor hallucis*

ANNOTATION KEY
Bold text indicates active muscles
Gray text indicates stabilizing muscles
* indicates deep muscles

SOLEUS STRETCH

The calf soleus stretch specifically targets the soleus muscles with a bend of the knee. This stretch improves flexibility and can also improve running speed.

BEST FOR

- soleus
- gastrocnemius

① Stand with one foot about one stride length back, knee bent.

② Bring the other foot forward and bend at the knee.

③ Keeping both heels on the ground, lean into the stretch as you bend your back knee. Once you feel the stretch, hold the position for fifteen seconds. Repeat stretch three times. Switch legs and repeat sequence three times.

DO IT RIGHT

LOOK FOR
- Your chest to remain upright as you lean into the stretch.

AVOID
- Allowing your ankles to rise off the ground.

gastrocnemius

soleus

peroneus longus

flexor hallucis longus

ANNOTATION KEY
Bold text indicates active muscles
Gray text indicates stabilizing muscles
* indicates deep muscles

PIRIFORMIS STRETCH

STRETCHES

The piriformis is a small muscle sandwiched between the glutes. By lying on the mat and distributing your weight evenly, you can obtain an effective, controlled stretch.

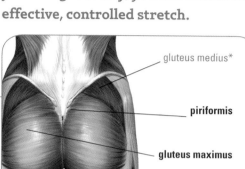

gluteus medius*

piriformis

gluteus maximus

vastus lateralis

ANNOTATION KEY
Bold text indicates active muscles
Gray text indicates stabilizing muscles
* indicates deep muscles

DO IT RIGHT

LOOK FOR
• Relaxing your hips so that you can go deeper into the stretch.
• Pulling your knee toward your chest slowly.

❶ Lie on your back with your knees bent.

❷ Bring one ankle over the opposite knee, resting it on your thigh. Place both hands around the thigh of the leg that is on the ground.

❸ Gently pull your thigh toward your chest until you feel the stretch in your buttocks. Hold for fifteen seconds and switch sides. Repeat sequence on opposite leg.

BEST FOR

• piriformis
• gluteus maximus
• gluteus medius

LUMBAR STRETCH

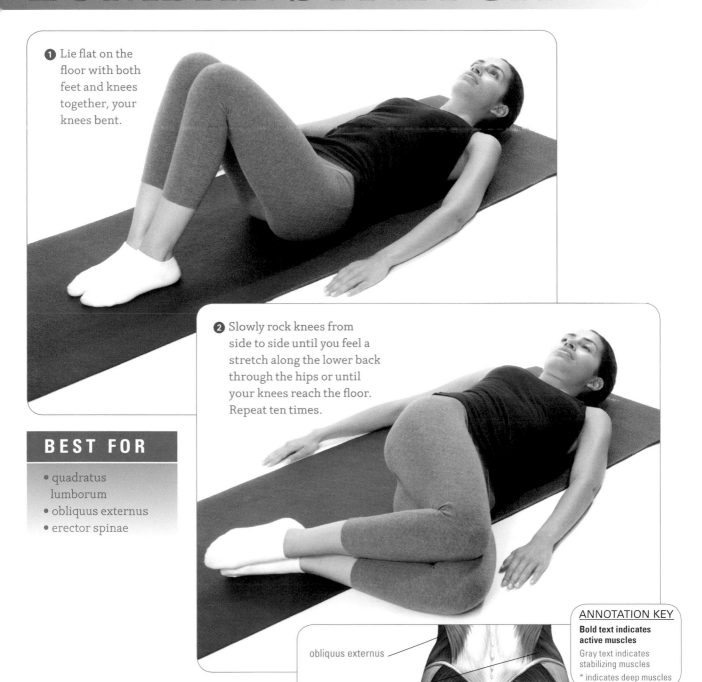

1 Lie flat on the floor with both feet and knees together, your knees bent.

2 Slowly rock knees from side to side until you feel a stretch along the lower back through the hips or until your knees reach the floor. Repeat ten times.

BEST FOR

- quadratus lumborum
- obliquus externus
- erector spinae

Use this stretch to open up your back and increase flexibility in an otherwise hard-to-reach area. If your knees can't reach the floor, try to get them as close as possible.

ANNOTATION KEY

Bold text indicates active muscles
Gray text indicates stabilizing muscles
* indicates deep muscles

obliquus externus

quadratus lumborum

gluteus medius*

erector spinae

SPINE STRETCH I

STRETCHES

This stretch increases the length and flexibility of the spine, an important aim of almost all of the exercises in this book. Make sure that the shoulders stay on the mat for the duration of the stretch.

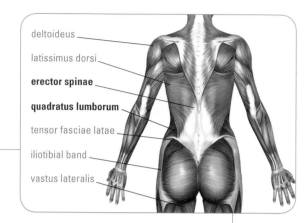

deltoideus
latissimus dorsi
erector spinae
quadratus lumborum
tensor fasciae latae
iliotibial band
vastus lateralis

ANNOTATION KEY
Bold text indicates active muscles
Gray text indicates stabilizing muscles
* indicates deep muscles

❶ Lie on your back with one leg straight and the other bent, placing the foot of your bent leg on your shin.

BEST FOR

- quadratus lumborum
- erector spinae
- vastus lateralis
- iliotibial band
- tensor fasciae latae

❷ Keeping both shoulders on the floor, slowly bring your bent leg across your body until you feel the stretch in the area between your lower back and hips. Stretch only as far as your shoulders will allow without one rising from the floor.

DO IT RIGHT

LOOK FOR
- Relaxing in your lower back.

AVOID
- Allowing your shoulders to come off the mat.

❸ Hold for fifteen seconds and repeat sequence three times on each side.

TRICEPS STRETCH

1. Standing, raise one arm and bend it behind your head.

2. Keeping your shoulders relaxed, gently pull on the raised elbow with your opposite hand.

3. Continue to pull on your elbow until you feel the stretch in your lower shoulder. Hold for fifteen seconds and repeat three times on each arm.

This simple stretch is key for any exercise that targets the upper body or for positions that rely on arm strength and stability, such as the plank position.

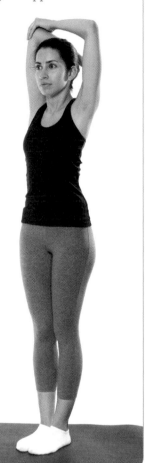

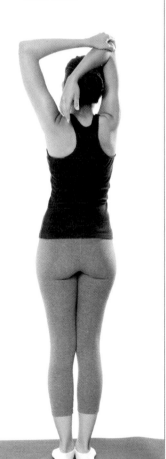

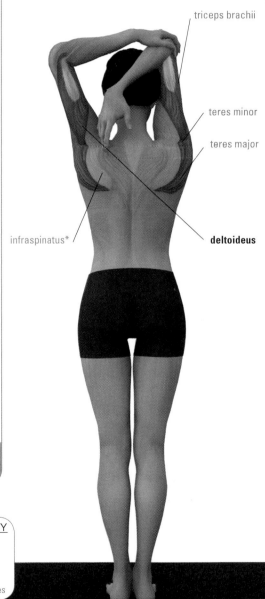

triceps brachii

teres minor

teres major

deltoideus

infraspinatus*

BEST FOR

- deltoideus
- infraspinatus
- teres major
- teres minor

ANNOTATION KEY
Bold text indicates active muscles
Gray text indicates stabilizing muscles
* indicates deep muscles

LATISSIMUS DORSI

STRETCHES

① Clasp your hands together above your head.

② Reach your hands outward as you make a circular pattern with your torso.

③ Slowly make a full circle. Repeat sequence three times in each direction.

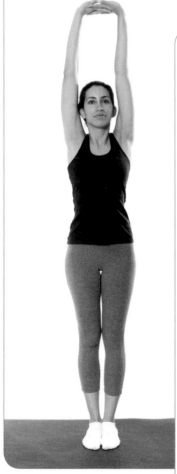

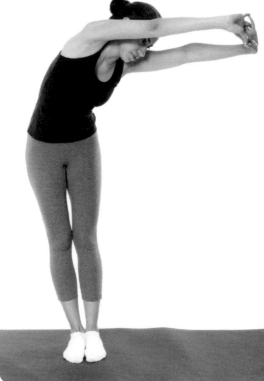

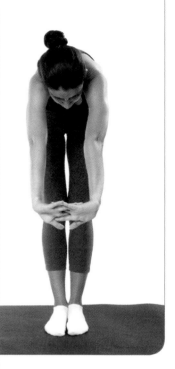

BEST FOR

- latissimus dorsi
- obliquus internus

STRETCH

The latissimus dorsi is a broad muscle that stretches from the back of the shoulder to the center of the spine. Stretching this muscle is often overlooked, but it is important in easing tension often caused by bad posture.

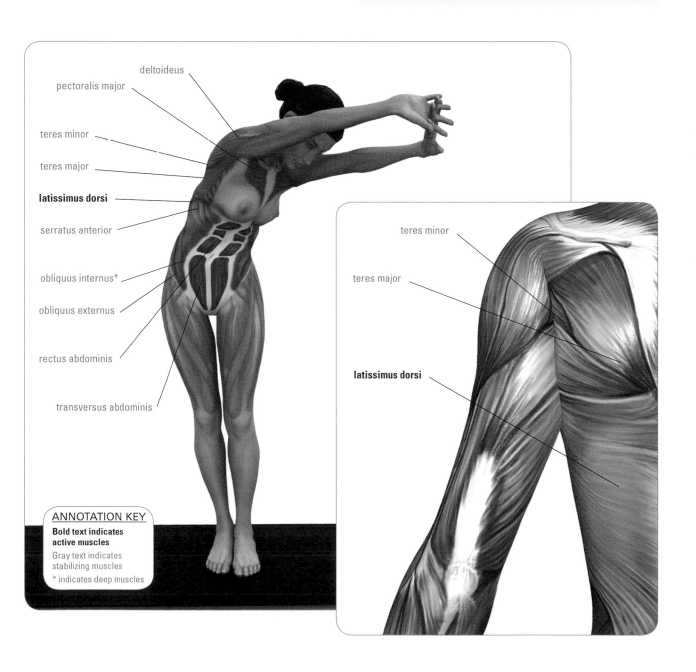

deltoideus

pectoralis major

teres minor

teres major

latissimus dorsi

serratus anterior

obliquus internus*

obliquus externus

rectus abdominis

transversus abdominis

teres minor

teres major

latissimus dorsi

ANNOTATION KEY
Bold text indicates active muscles
Gray text indicates stabilizing muscles
* indicates deep muscles

NECK FLEXION

STRETCHES

The neck is as important as the spine in many Pilates exercises. The neck flexion stretch will aid in keeping the neck long and flexible, protecting against pain and eliminating unnecessary tension.

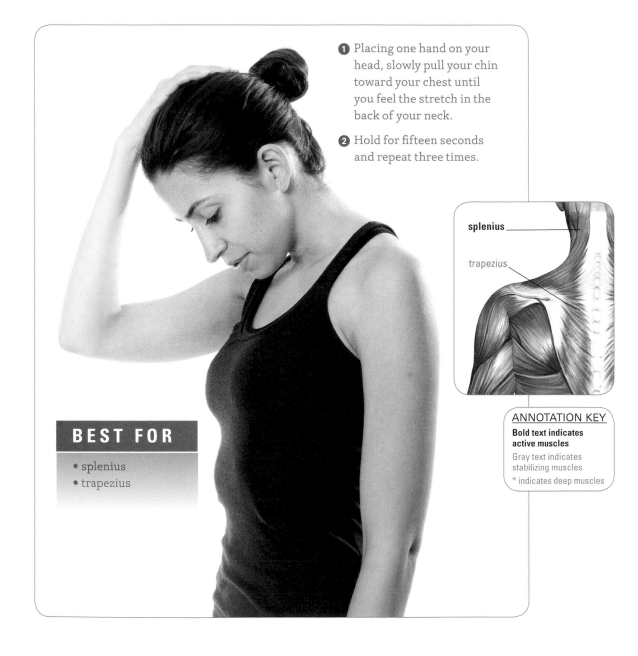

① Placing one hand on your head, slowly pull your chin toward your chest until you feel the stretch in the back of your neck.

② Hold for fifteen seconds and repeat three times.

splenius

trapezius

BEST FOR
• splenius
• trapezius

ANNOTATION KEY
Bold text indicates active muscles
Gray text indicates stabilizing muscles
* indicates deep muscles

SIDE-BEND STRETCH

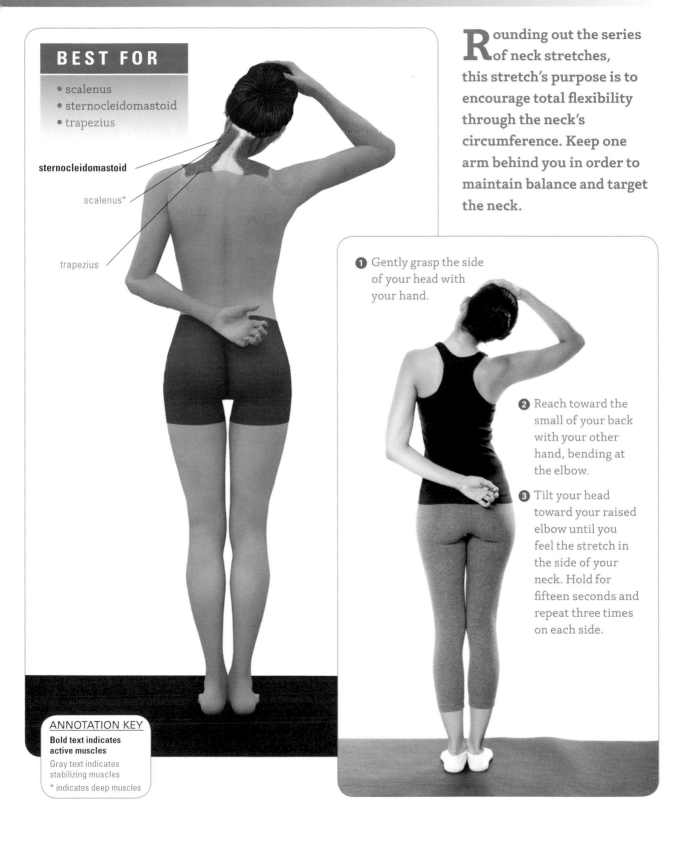

BEST FOR
- scalenus
- sternocleidomastoid
- trapezius

sternocleidomastoid

scalenus*

trapezius

Rounding out the series of neck stretches, this stretch's purpose is to encourage total flexibility through the neck's circumference. Keep one arm behind you in order to maintain balance and target the neck.

➊ Gently grasp the side of your head with your hand.

➋ Reach toward the small of your back with your other hand, bending at the elbow.

➌ Tilt your head toward your raised elbow until you feel the stretch in the side of your neck. Hold for fifteen seconds and repeat three times on each side.

ANNOTATION KEY
Bold text indicates active muscles
Gray text indicates stabilizing muscles
* indicates deep muscles

THE EXERCISES

The exercises in this book are broken down into three skill levels: Beginner, Intermediate, and Advanced. If you're just beginning your exploration of Pilates, start with the Beginner exercises after you've mastered the warm-up and cool-down stretches. For those with previous Pilates training, you may be comfortable skipping ahead to the Intermediate or Advanced sections—much of what you have already mastered will provide a good foundation for these more challenging exercises.

Pay attention to the specific tips and suggestions that accompany each exercise. It's a good idea to familiarize yourself with this information before you attempt any of the exercises—that way you'll know exactly what to look for, what to avoid, and—if you suffer from pain or injury—when to avoid an exercise entirely.

The progression of these sections serves to reinforce the layered, repetitive structure of Pilates—you'll start by isolating and exercising singular muscles in the Beginner section, and engage several groups of muscles at once as the exercises become more challenging. The goal for all of these exercises remains the same, though—better control of your body through flexibility, muscle length, and repetition.

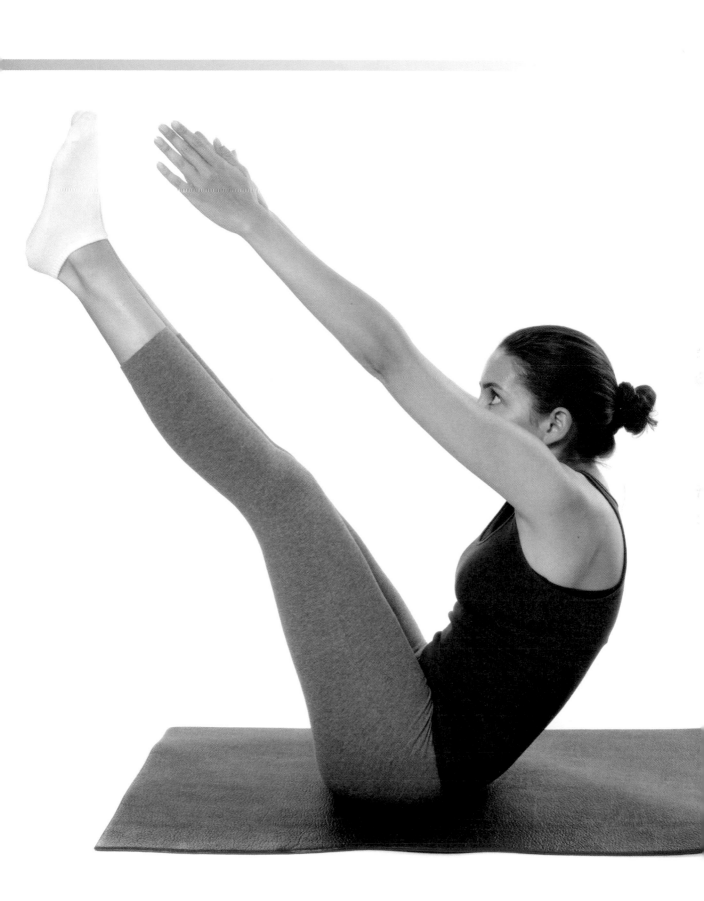

HALF CURL

BEGINNER

The Half Curl is a simple abdominal exercise that strengthens your core muscles, protecting your back while increasing muscle tone.

BEST FOR

- rectus abdominis
- latissimus dorsi
- pectoralis major
- sternohyoid
- sternocleidomastoid
- deltoideus
- biceps brachii
- triceps brachii

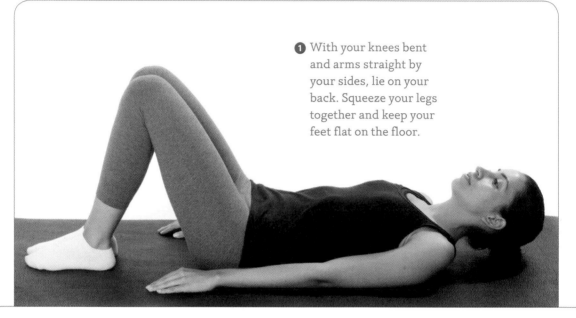

1 With your knees bent and arms straight by your sides, lie on your back. Squeeze your legs together and keep your feet flat on the floor.

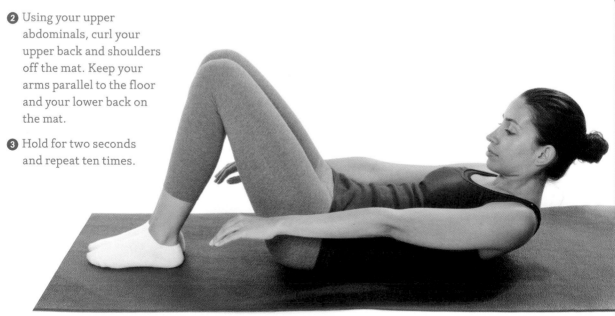

2 Using your upper abdominals, curl your upper back and shoulders off the mat. Keep your arms parallel to the floor and your lower back on the mat.

3 Hold for two seconds and repeat ten times.

DO IT RIGHT

LOOK FOR
- Keeping your arms parallel to the floor.

AVOID
- Curling your neck too far forward.
- Allowing your feet to raise off the floor.

ANNOTATION KEY
Bold text indicates active muscles
Gray text indicates stabilizing muscles
* indicates deep muscles

biceps brachii
deltoideus
pectoralis major
rectus abdominis
obliquus externus
extensor digitorum
brachioradialis
sternocleidomastoideus
triceps brachii
sternohyoid

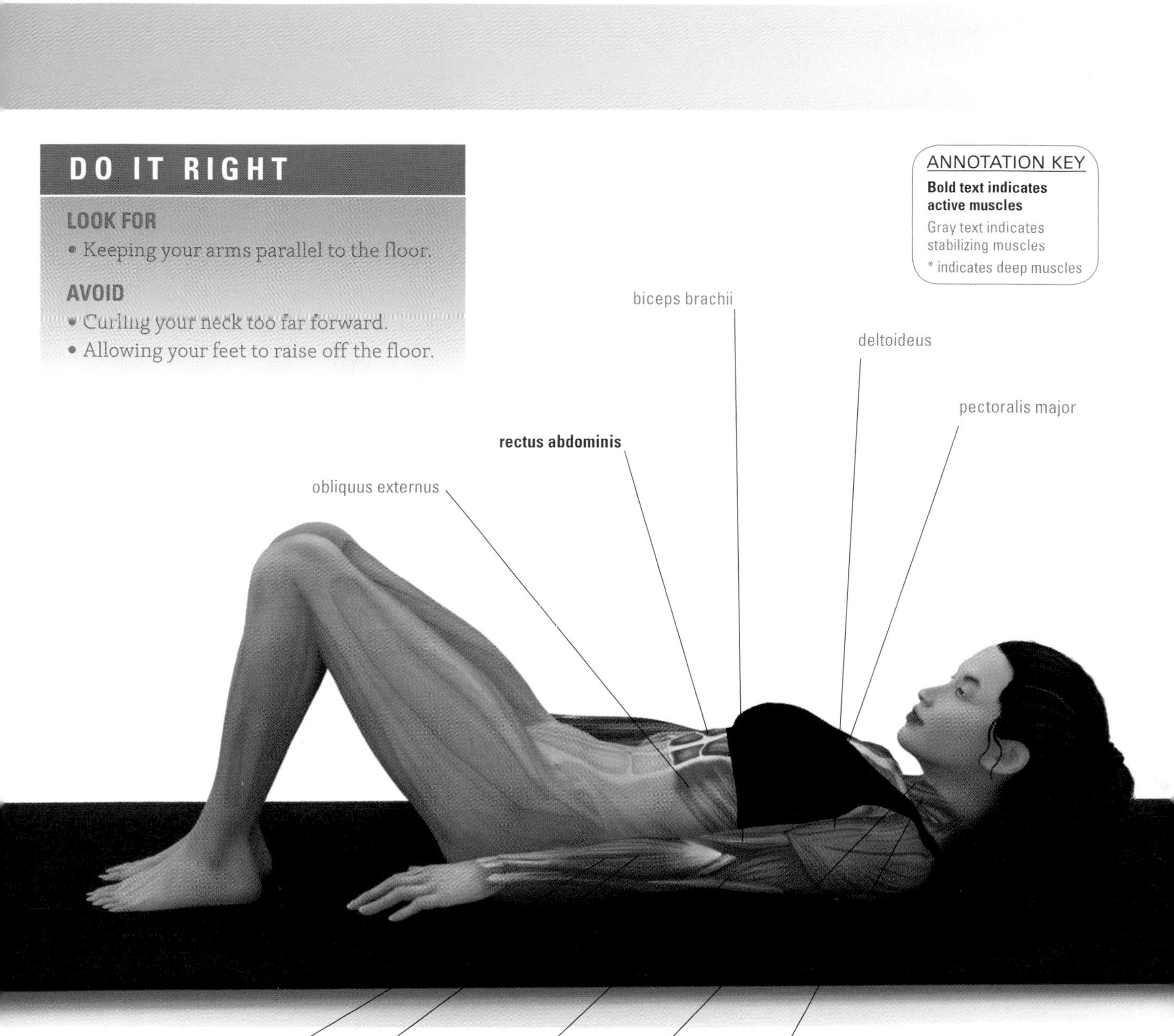

QUICK GUIDE

TARGET
- Upper abdominal muscles

BENEFITS
- Strengthens core muscles
- Increases abdominal endurance

NOT ADVISABLE IF YOU HAVE
- Cervical spine issues

TINY STEPS

Oftentimes, those who want to get in shape put such an emphasis on working the upper abdominal muscles while exercising that they tend to ignore the harder-to-reach lower abdominals.

The Tiny Steps exercise works these muscles by adding leg movement, which helps to develop stability, protects the lower back, and strengthens all of the muscles surrounding the hips.

❶ With your knees bent and feet flat on floor, lie on your back in supine position.

❷ Place your hands on your hip bones to feel if you are moving your hips from side to side.

❸ Exhaling, raise your right knee to your chest while pulling your navel toward your spine. Inhale and hold position.

❹ Exhale again, continuing to pull your navel toward your spine. Lower your right leg onto the mat while controlling any movement in your hips.

QUICK GUIDE

TARGET
• Lower abdominal muscles

BENEFITS
• Develops lower abdominal stability, protecting your hips and lower back

NOT ADVISABLE IF YOU HAVE
• Sharp lower back pain that radiates down the legs

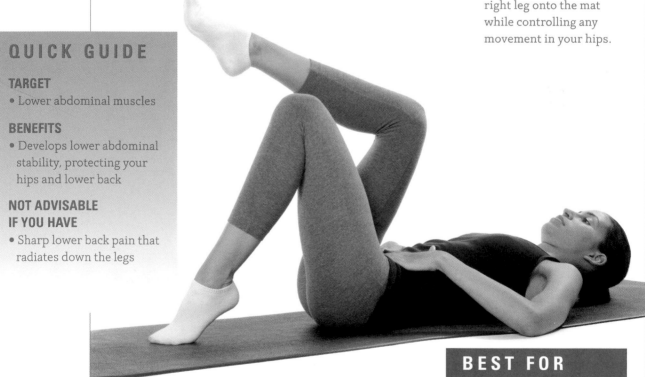

BEST FOR

• rectus abdominis
• rectus femoris
• gluteus maximus
• tensor fasciae latae
• transversus abdominis
• obliquus internus

5 Alternate legs to complete the full movement. Repeat six to eight times.

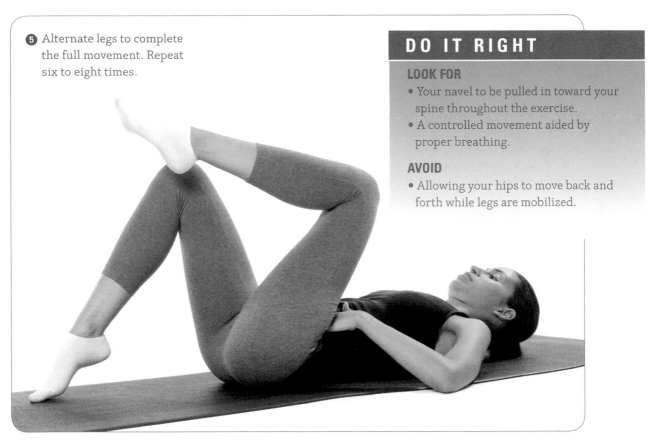

DO IT RIGHT

LOOK FOR
- Your navel to be pulled in toward your spine throughout the exercise.
- A controlled movement aided by proper breathing.

AVOID
- Allowing your hips to move back and forth while legs are mobilized.

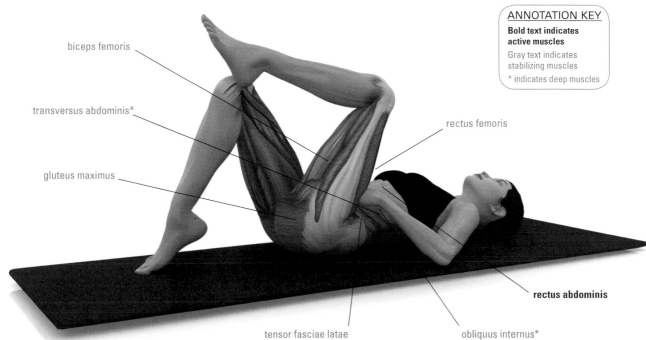

ANNOTATION KEY
Bold text indicates active muscles
Gray text indicates stabilizing muscles
* indicates deep muscles

biceps femoris

transversus abdominis*

gluteus maximus

rectus femoris

rectus abdominis

tensor fasciae latae

obliquus internus*

SIDE LEG LIFT PREP

BEGINNER

Another core stability exercise, the Side Leg Lift Prep helps tone and strengthen the leg and abdominal muscles. The Side Leg Lift Prep is an excellent introduction exercise that works as a base for more advanced Pilates movements.

DO IT RIGHT

LOOK FOR
• Your outside hand to be placed on the ankle of your bent leg, and your inside hand to be placed on your bent knee.
• The top of your sternum and your head to be lifted forward.

AVOID
• Allowing your lower back to come off the floor; use abdominals to stabilize your core while switching legs.

❶ Lie on your right side on the back edge of the mat. Prop your head up with your left hand, resting on your elbow. Place your right hand in front of your torso, keeping your chest lifted and your neck elongated.

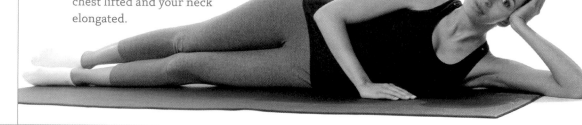

QUICK GUIDE

TARGET
• Pelvic stabilizer muscles
• Oblique abdominal muscles

BENEFITS
• Tones and lengthens the legs and torso
• Strengthens core muscles

NOT ADVISABLE IF YOU HAVE
• Neck issues

❷ Draw in your abdominals, pulling your navel toward your spine. Lift both legs up in the air, squeezing them tightly.

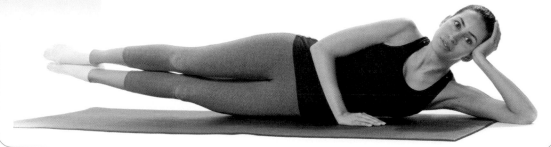

3 Without moving your torso or hips, bring your legs forward and lower them to the front edge of the mat with control. Your legs and torso should make a 45-degree angle with the mat. Your hips and shoulders should be aligned.

4 Squeezing your abdominals and legs, lift your legs and return to the original position. Repeat five to six times on each side.

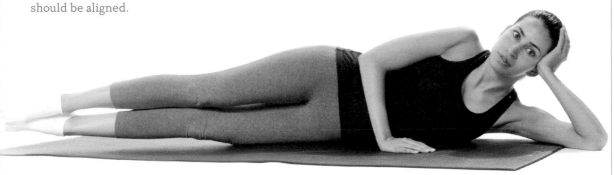

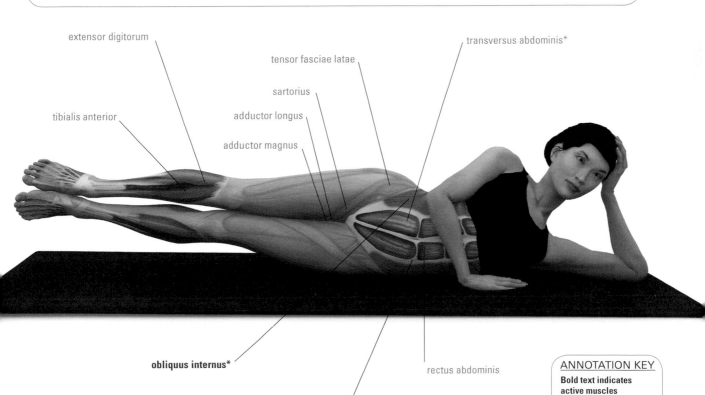

extensor digitorum

tensor fasciae latae

transversus abdominis*

sartorius

tibialis anterior

adductor longus

adductor magnus

obliquus internus*

rectus abdominis

obliquus externus

ANNOTATION KEY
Bold text indicates active muscles
Gray text indicates stabilizing muscles
* indicates deep muscles

ROLLING LIKE A BALL

BEGINNER

The Rolling Like a Ball exercise focuses on balance and control, spinal articulation, and stretching. It also feels good, giving you a back massage as you exercise.

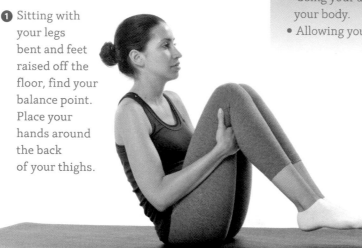

❶ Sitting with your legs bent and feet raised off the floor, find your balance point. Place your hands around the back of your thighs.

QUICK GUIDE

TARGET
• Abdominal muscles

BENEFITS
• Massages back muscles
• Enhances abdominal control

NOT ADVISABLE IF YOU HAVE
• Neck issues

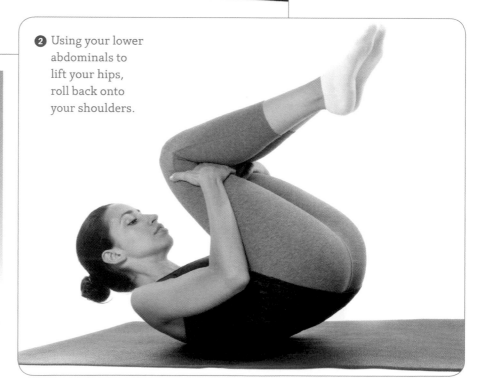

❷ Using your lower abdominals to lift your hips, roll back onto your shoulders.

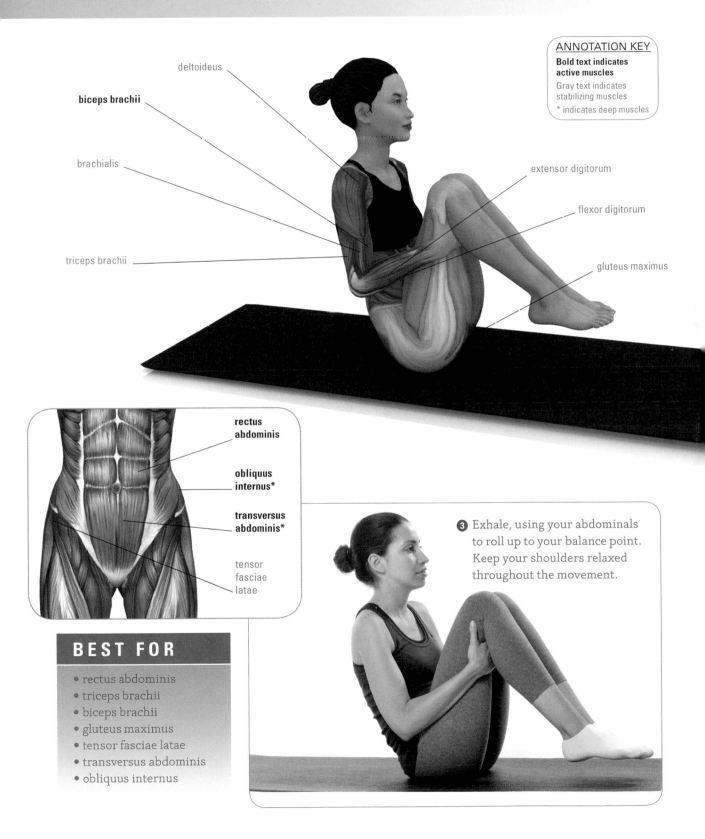

deltoideus

biceps brachii

brachialis

triceps brachii

extensor digitorum

flexor digitorum

gluteus maximus

**rectus
abdominis**

**obliquus
internus***

**transversus
abdominis***

tensor
fasciae
latae

BEST FOR

- rectus abdominis
- triceps brachii
- biceps brachii
- gluteus maximus
- tensor fasciae latae
- transversus abdominis
- obliquus internus

❸ Exhale, using your abdominals
to roll up to your balance point.
Keep your shoulders relaxed
throughout the movement.

SPINE STRETCH II

BEGINNER

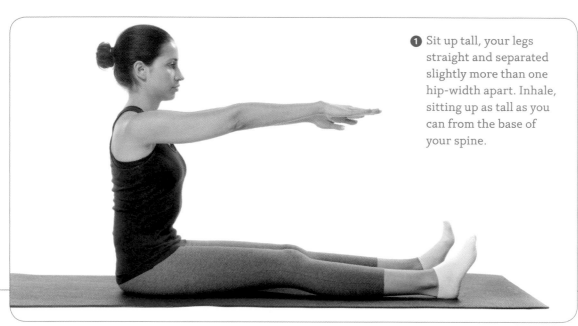

1. Sit up tall, your legs straight and separated slightly more than one hip-width apart. Inhale, sitting up as tall as you can from the base of your spine.

BEST FOR

- gluteus maximus
- gluteus medius
- biceps femoris
- semitendinosus
- latissimus dorsi
- obliquus internus

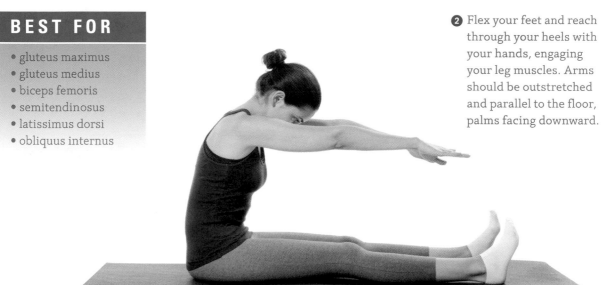

2. Flex your feet and reach through your heels with your hands, engaging your leg muscles. Arms should be outstretched and parallel to the floor, palms facing downward.

The Spine Stretch is another exercise involving the forward curling of the back. The spine stretch increases flexibility, helping you prevent injuries and gain better posture.

DO IT RIGHT

LOOK FOR
- Sitting high on your sit bones.
- Articulating one vertebra at a time as you stretch forward and roll back up.

❸ Exhale, rounding your back into a C curve by pulling in your ribs and stomach. Roll your head downward, stretching your neck.

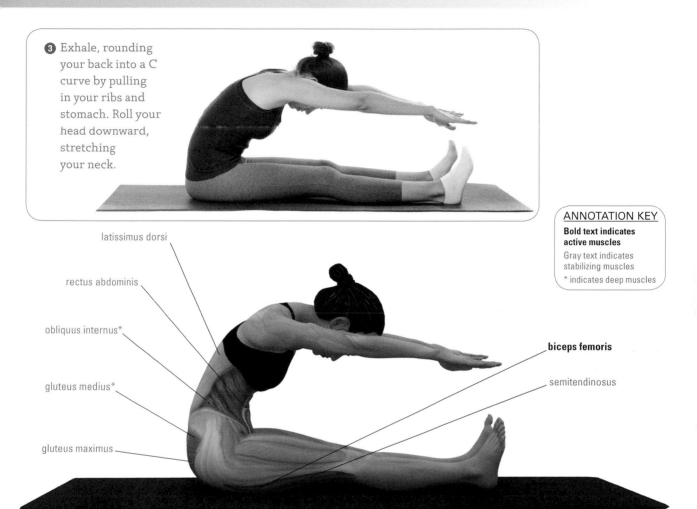

latissimus dorsi

rectus abdominis

obliquus internus*

gluteus medius*

gluteus maximus

biceps femoris

semitendinosus

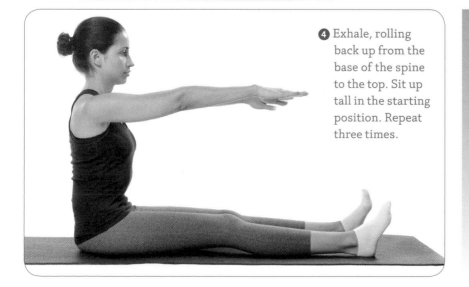

❹ Exhale, rolling back up from the base of the spine to the top. Sit up tall in the starting position. Repeat three times.

QUICK GUIDE

TARGET
• Hip and hamstring flexibility

BENEFITS
• A great stretch for the entire spine, especially the neck and upper back

NOT ADVISABLE IF YOU HAVE
• Stress on the lower back. For very tight hamstrings, use a folded towel to sit on during the exercise.

SPINE TWIST

BEGINNER

1 Sit on mat, with back straight. Extend legs in front of you, slightly more than one hip-width apart.

2 Inhale, lifting yourself as tall as you can from the base of your spine. Think of grounding your hips into the floor.

The Spine Twist is one of the best ways to increase the range of motion in your upper body. This exercise helps stretch the back and torso while maintaining a central vertical axis through the body.

BEST FOR

- biceps femoris
- gluteus maximus
- tensor fasciae latae
- transversus abdominis
- obliquus externus
- latissimus dorsi
- teres major
- quadratus lumborum
- deltoideus
- rectus femoris

3 Exhale, lifting up and out of your hips as you pull in your lower abdominals. Twist from your waist to the left, keeping your hips square and grounded.

4 Inhale, and return to the center.

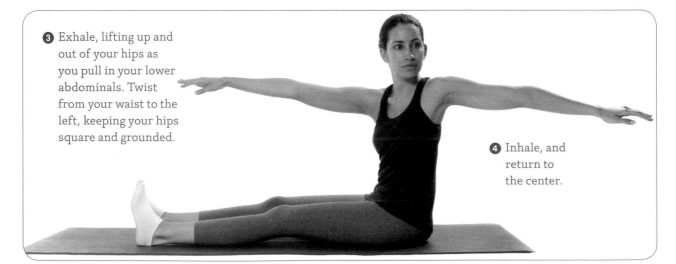

DO IT RIGHT

LOOK FOR
- Your torso to rotate along the central axis of your body.
- Your arms to remain parallel to the floor.

AVOID
- Allowing your hips to rise off the floor.

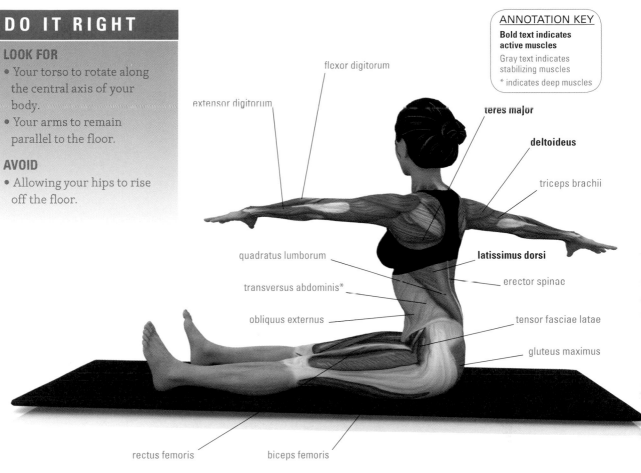

flexor digitorum

extensor digitorum

teres major

deltoideus

triceps brachii

quadratus lumborum

latissimus dorsi

erector spinae

transversus abdominis*

obliquus externus

tensor fasciae latae

gluteus maximus

rectus femoris

biceps femoris

QUICK GUIDE

TARGET
- Back flexibility

BENEFITS
- Strengthens and lengthens the torso

NOT ADVISABLE IF YOU HAVE
- Back pain. If your hamstrings are too tight to sit up straight, place a towel under your buttocks and bend your knees slightly.

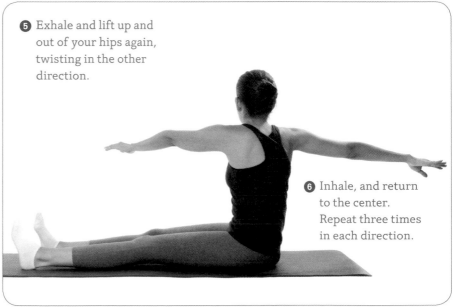

5 Exhale and lift up and out of your hips again, twisting in the other direction.

6 Inhale, and return to the center. Repeat three times in each direction.

ROLL-DOWN

The Roll-down enables you to transition into other exercises, improving both abdominal strength and stability simultaneously.

BEST FOR

- rectus abdominis
- tensor fasciae latae
- obliquus internus
- obliquus externus
- transversus abdominis

1 While seated, bend your knees and place your feet flat on the floor. Inhale while sitting up as tall as you can, lengthening your spine.

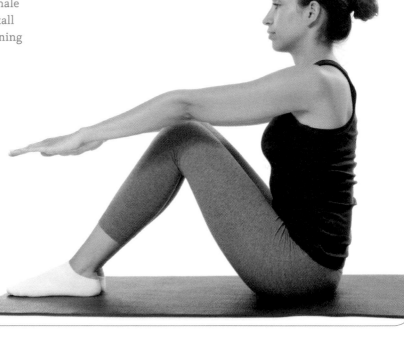

DO IT RIGHT

LOOK FOR
- Your outside hand to be placed on the ankle of your bent leg, and your inside hand to be placed on your bent knee.
- The top of your sternum and your head to be lifted forward.

AVOID
- Allowing your lower back to come off the floor; use abdominals to stabilize core while switching legs.

2 Exhale, pulling your navel toward your spine, creating a C curve in your back. Begin rolling backward down your spine, tucking your tailbone beneath you. Your arms should remain outstretched and parallel in front of you.

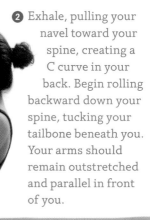

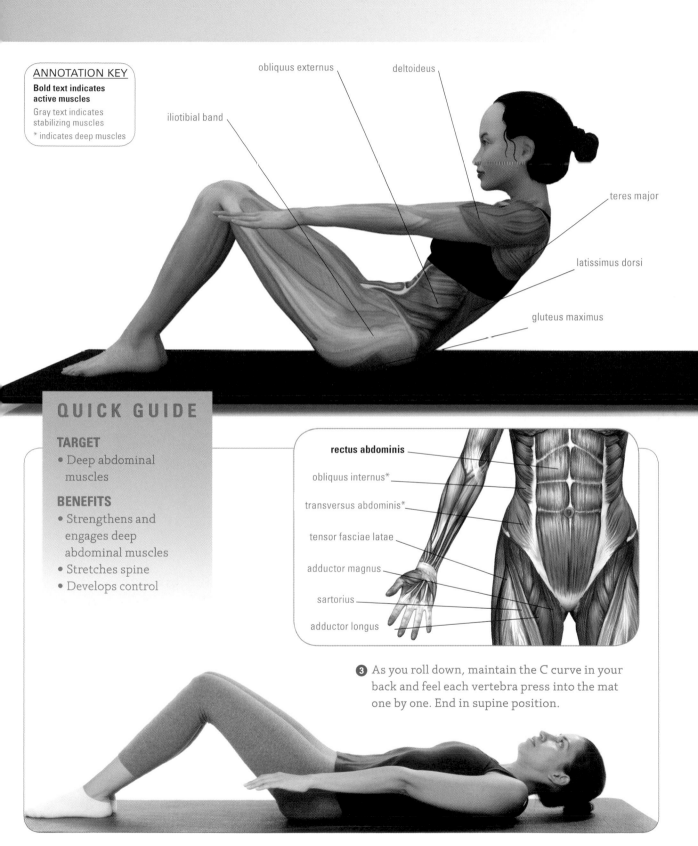

ANNOTATION KEY
**Bold text indicates
active muscles**
Gray text indicates
stabilizing muscles
* indicates deep muscles

obliquus externus

deltoideus

iliotibial band

teres major

latissimus dorsi

gluteus maximus

QUICK GUIDE

TARGET
• Deep abdominal
  muscles

BENEFITS
• Strengthens and
  engages deep
  abdominal muscles
• Stretches spine
• Develops control

rectus abdominis

obliquus internus*

transversus abdominis*

tensor fasciae latae

adductor magnus

sartorius

adductor longus

❸ As you roll down, maintain the C curve in your
back and feel each vertebra press into the mat
one by one. End in supine position.

BRIDGE I

BEGINNER

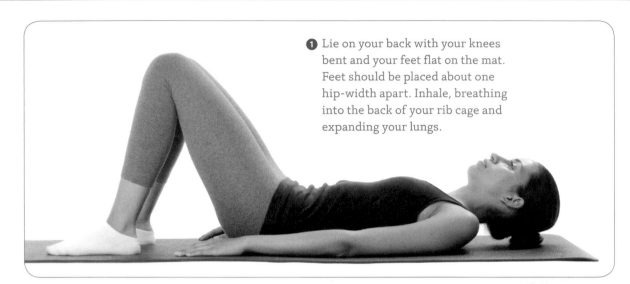

1 Lie on your back with your knees bent and your feet flat on the mat. Feet should be placed about one hip-width apart. Inhale, breathing into the back of your rib cage and expanding your lungs.

Bridging is the perfect exercise for toning the legs and buttocks. Exercising these muscles while stabilizing the torso also benefits the lower back by both strengthening weak areas and protecting it from future injury.

BEST FOR

- gluteus maximus
- biceps femoris
- rectus femoris
- rectus abdominis
- tensor fasciae latae
- transversus abdominis
- obliquus internus

2 Exhale and press your feet into the mat and squeeze your buttocks together, raising your hips until your body makes a straight line from your shoulders to your knees.

3 Inhale and hold the position.

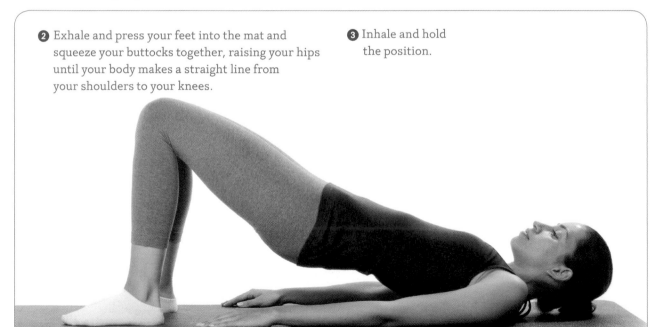

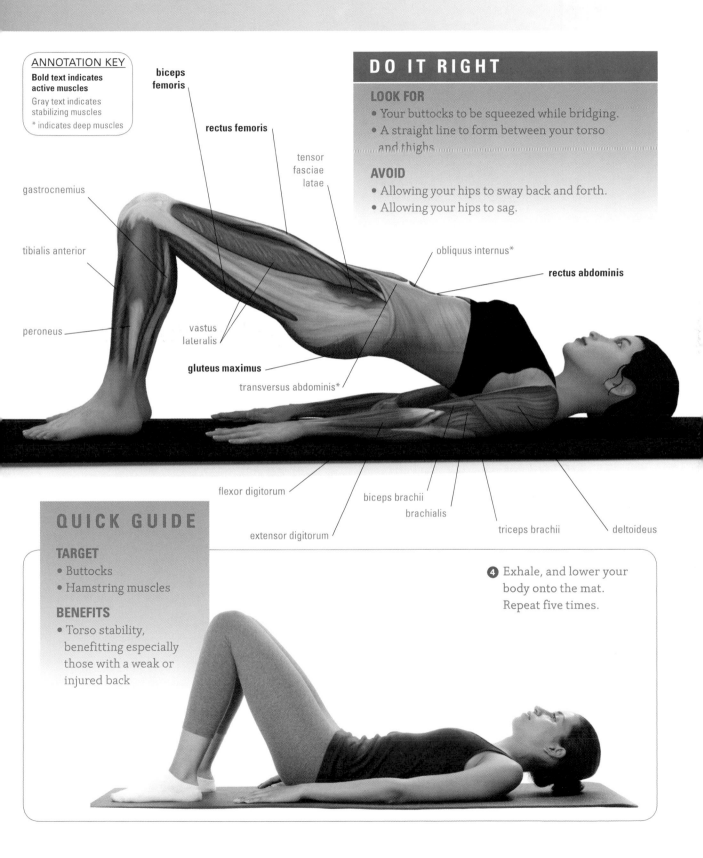

ANNOTATION KEY
**Bold text indicates
active muscles**
Gray text indicates
stabilizing muscles
* indicates deep muscles

**biceps
femoris**

rectus femoris

tensor
fasciae
latae

gastrocnemius

tibialis anterior

peroneus

vastus
lateralis

gluteus maximus

transversus abdominis*

obliquus internus*

rectus abdominis

flexor digitorum

extensor digitorum

biceps brachii

brachialis

triceps brachii

deltoideus

DO IT RIGHT

LOOK FOR
• Your buttocks to be squeezed while bridging.
• A straight line to form between your torso
and thighs.

AVOID
• Allowing your hips to sway back and forth.
• Allowing your hips to sag.

QUICK GUIDE

TARGET
• Buttocks
• Hamstring muscles

BENEFITS
• Torso stability,
benefitting especially
those with a weak or
injured back

❹ Exhale, and lower your
body onto the mat.
Repeat five times.

SINGLE-LEG CIRCLES

BEGINNER

Single-leg Circles are perfect for developing abdominal control. Working one side at a time allows you to focus on multiple leg and abdominal muscles.

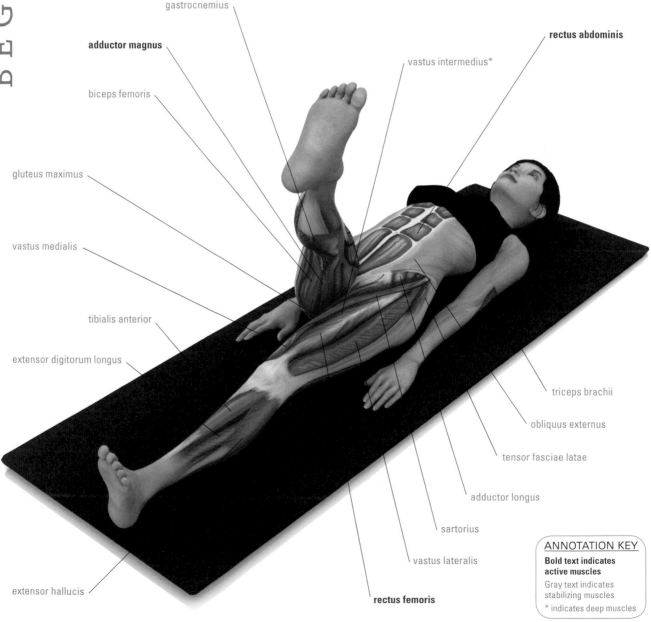

gastrocnemius

adductor magnus

biceps femoris

gluteus maximus

vastus medialis

tibialis anterior

extensor digitorum longus

extensor hallucis

vastus intermedius*

rectus abdominis

triceps brachii

obliquus externus

tensor fasciae latae

adductor longus

sartorius

vastus lateralis

rectus femoris

ANNOTATION KEY

Bold text indicates active muscles

Gray text indicates stabilizing muscles

* indicates deep muscles

① Lie flat on the floor with both legs and arms extended.

② Begin by bending your right knee toward your chest, and then straighten your leg up in the air. Anchor the rest of your body to the mat, straightening both knees and pressing your shoulders back and down.

③ Cross your raised leg up and over your body, aiming for your left shoulder. Continue making a circle with the raised leg and return to the center.

Add an emphasis to the motion by pausing at the top between repetitions.

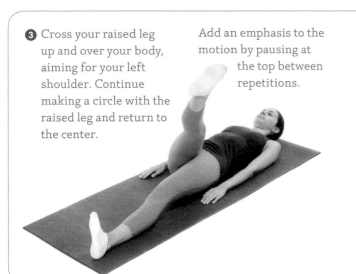

④ Switch directions and repeat. Repeat with other leg. Complete full movement five to eight times.

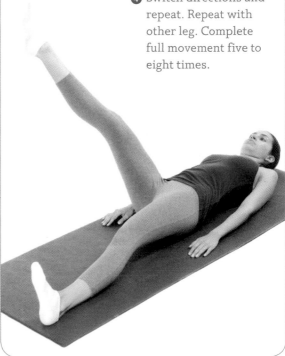

DO IT RIGHT

LOOK FOR
• Maintaining stability in your hips and torso while your legs are mobilized.
• Elongating your leg from your hip through your foot.

THE HUNDRED I

BEGINNER

The Hundred is a perfect warm-up for the lungs and abdominal muscles. It helps increase endurance while building proper breathing techniques.

1 Lie on your back with your feet flat on the floor and squeeze your inner thighs together.

2 Inhale, reaching your arms into the air with your palms facing forward.

3 Exhale, bringing your arms toward the floor and lengthening the back of your neck with a gentle chin tuck (you can lift your head at this point if keeping it down is too easy). Gently pulse your arms up and down in a small percussive motion as if you are slapping water, simultaneously pushing down and back with your shoulders.

4 Inhale deeply for five beats while maintaining the rhythm with your arms, focusing on drawing in the lower abdominals more deeply. Gently force exhalation using your abdominal muscles for an additional five beats.

5 Hold the position and pulse your arms for ten full breaths for a total of one hundred beats.

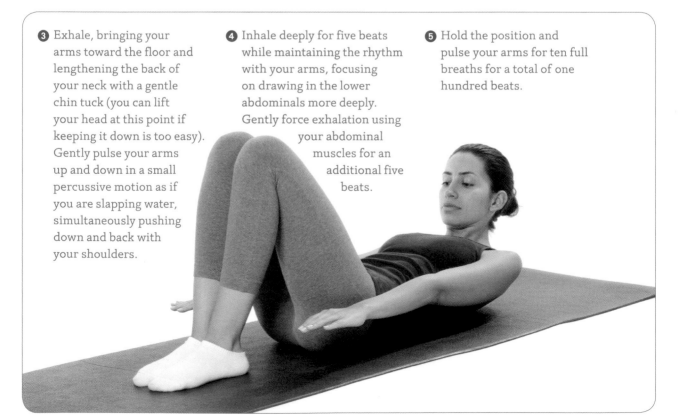

DO IT RIGHT

LOOK FOR
- Your breathing to remain steady.
- Your abdominals to be pulled in toward your spine.

AVOID
- Allowing your lower back to arch while you pump your arms.

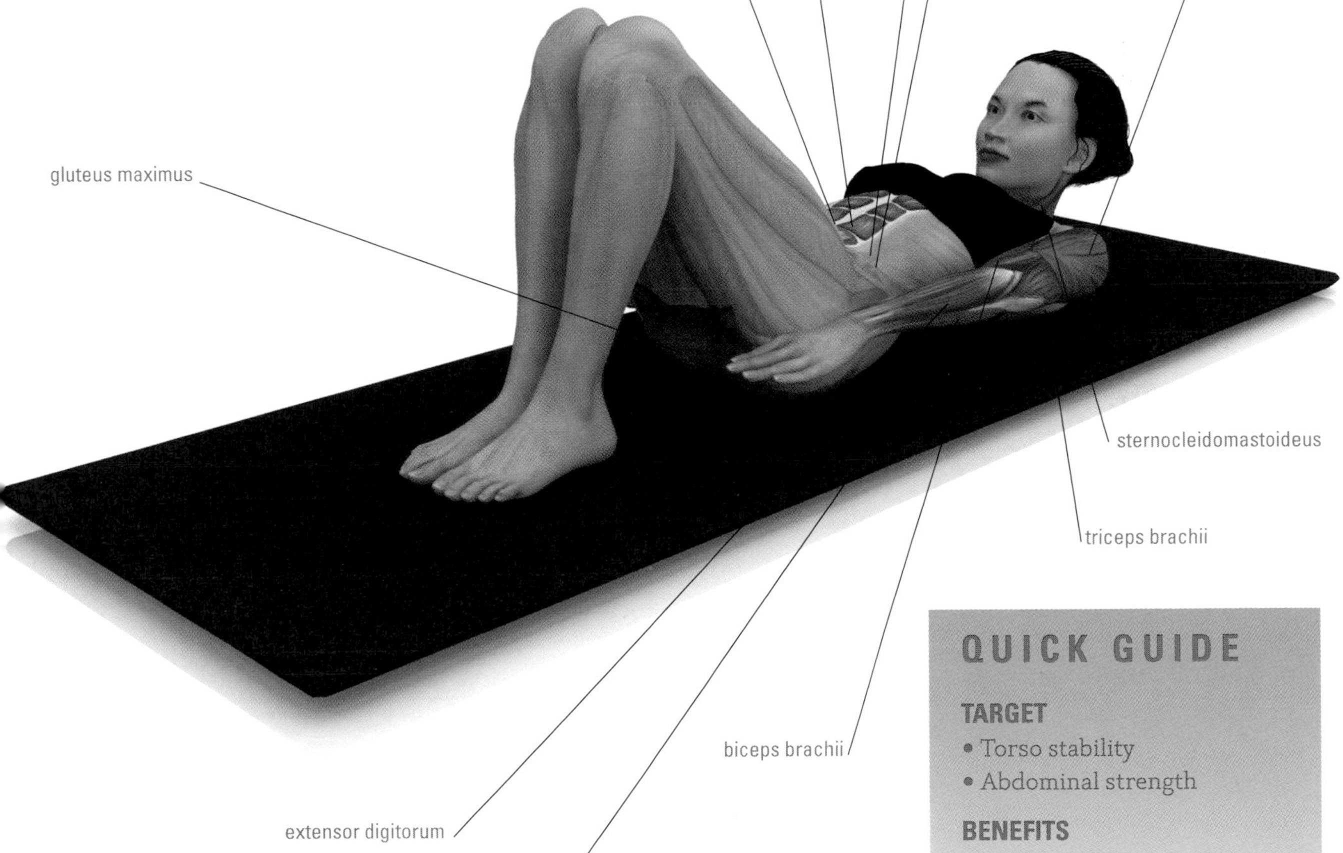

obliquus internus*

rectus abdominis

deltoideus

obliquus externus

transversus abdominis*

gluteus maximus

sternocleidomastoideus

triceps brachii

biceps brachii

extensor digitorum

flexor digitorum

QUICK GUIDE

TARGET
- Torso stability
- Abdominal strength

BENEFITS
- Warms up the muscles to increase blood flow

NOT ADVISABLE IF YOU HAVE
- Lower-back pain

ANNOTATION KEY
Bold text indicates active muscles
Gray text indicates stabilizing muscles
* indicates deep muscles

SINGLE-LEG STRETCH

BEGINNER

The Single-leg Stretch is a beginner exercise that targets the abdominal muscles and helps improve coordination.

BEST FOR

- rectus abdominis
- biceps femoris
- triceps brachii
- biceps brachii
- tibialis anterior
- tensor fasciae latae
- transversus abdominis
- obliquus internus

❶ Pull one knee to your chest and straighten your other leg, raising it about 45 degrees from the floor.

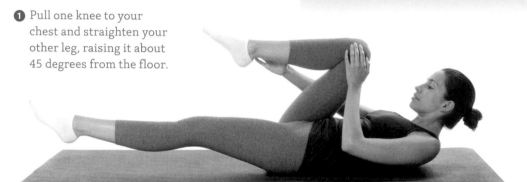

❷ Place your outside hand on the ankle of your bent leg, and your inside hand on the knee of your bent leg (this maintains proper alignment of leg).

ANNOTATION KEY

Bold text indicates active muscles

Gray text indicates stabilizing muscles

* indicates deep muscles

QUICK GUIDE

TARGET
- Torso stability
- Abdominals

BENEFITS
- Stabilizes core while extremities are in motion
- Strengthens abdominals

NOT ADVISABLE IF YOU HAVE
- Neck issues
- Lower-back pain

biceps femoris

rectus abdominis

triceps brachii

rectus femoris

biceps brachii

tibialis anterior

tensor fasciae latae

transversus abdominis*

obliquus internus

DO IT RIGHT

LOOK FOR
- Your outside hand to be placed on the ankle of your bent leg, and your inside hand to be placed on your bent knee.
- The top of your sternum and your head to be lifted forward.

AVOID
- Allowing your lower back to come off the floor; use abdominals to stabilize core while switching legs.

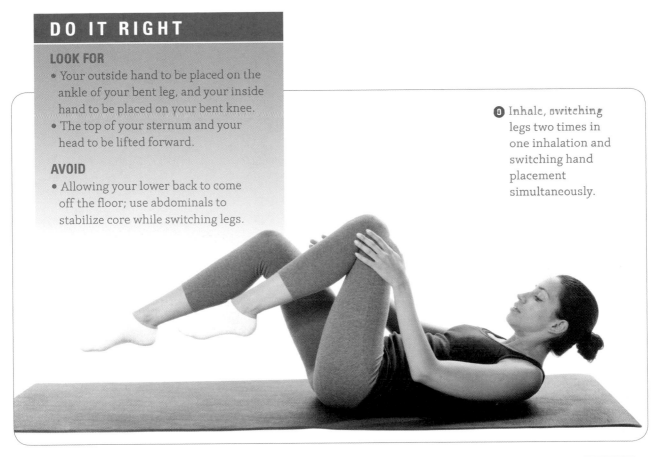

③ Inhale, switching legs two times in one inhalation and switching hand placement simultaneously.

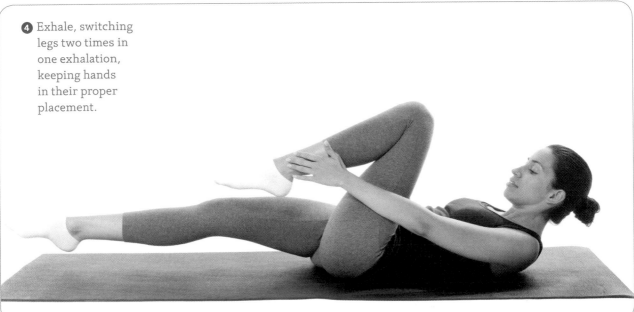

④ Exhale, switching legs two times in one exhalation, keeping hands in their proper placement.

DOUBLE-LEG STRETCH

BEGINNER

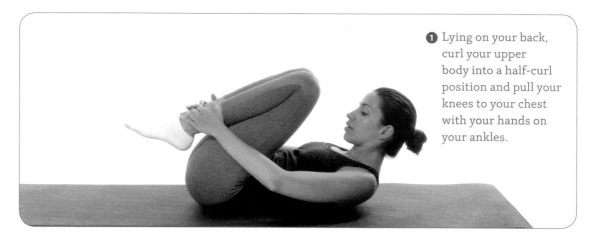

1 Lying on your back, curl your upper body into a half-curl position and pull your knees to your chest with your hands on your ankles.

The Double-leg Stretch takes the Single-leg Stretch a step further by bringing both legs into the body. This is slightly more challenging for the leg and abdominal muscles, and it also builds strength in the back.

BEST FOR

- rectus abdominis
- biceps femoris
- triceps brachii
- biceps brachii
- tibialis anterior
- tensor fasciae latae
- transversus abdominis
- obliquus internus
- rectus femoris

QUICK GUIDE

TARGET
- Abdominal muscles

BENEFITS
- Lengthens legs
- Strengthens abdominal muscles

NOT ADVISABLE IF YOU HAVE
- Lower-back pain

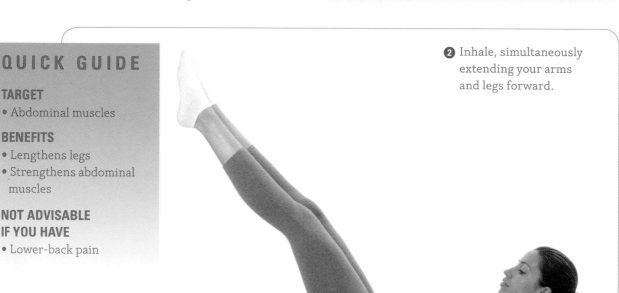

2 Inhale, simultaneously extending your arms and legs forward.

DO IT RIGHT

LOOK FOR
• Your head to be lifted off the mat with your neck elongated.

AVOID
• Allowing your lower back to come off the floor; use abdominals to stabilize core while legs are extended.

MODIFICATIONS

More Difficult: Instead of extending your arms forward during the inhalation, reach your arms behind your head while extending your legs.

ANNOTATION KEY
Bold text indicates active muscles
Gray text indicates stabilizing muscles
* indicates deep muscles

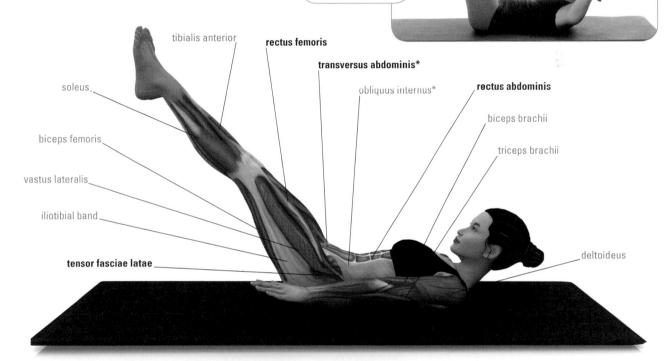

tibialis anterior
rectus femoris
transversus abdominis*
obliquus internus*
rectus abdominis
soleus
biceps femoris
vastus lateralis
iliotibial band
tensor fasciae latae
biceps brachii
triceps brachii
deltoideus

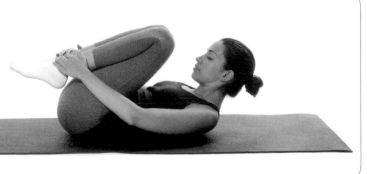

❸ Exhale while hugging your knees back into the center. Make sure you are keeping your upper body lifted off the mat. Repeat four times.

THE RISING SWAN

BEGINNER

1 Lie facedown with your forehead on the mat, arms bent, and elbows close to your sides with palms facing downward. Turn out your legs from the top of your hips and pull your inner thighs together.

2 Pull your navel off of the mat and toward the spine, simultaneously pressing your pubic bone into the mat. Squeeze your buttocks and inhale.

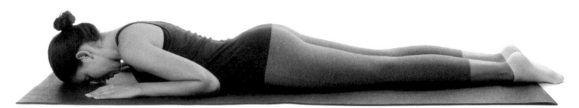

3 Exhale, scooping in your stomach while pressing through your hands to slowly rise from your upper back. Keep the back of your neck elongated and lift your head gently off the mat.

4 Inhale and hold the position, drawing your navel deeper into your spine and squeezing your buttocks, all the while keeping your legs in contact with the mat.

5 Exhale and return to starting position.

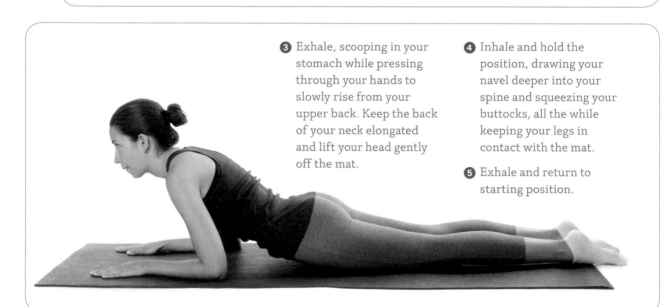

It is important to extend the back with an arching movement in order to equalize forward movement in the spine. The Rising Swan strengthens the back, neck, and buttocks while stabilizing the pelvis.

BEST FOR

- gluteus maximus
- biceps femoris
- rectus femoris
- deltoideus
- triceps brachii
- biceps brachii
- teres major
- latissimus dorsi
- quadratus lumborum
- tensor fasciae latae
- brachialis
- trapezius

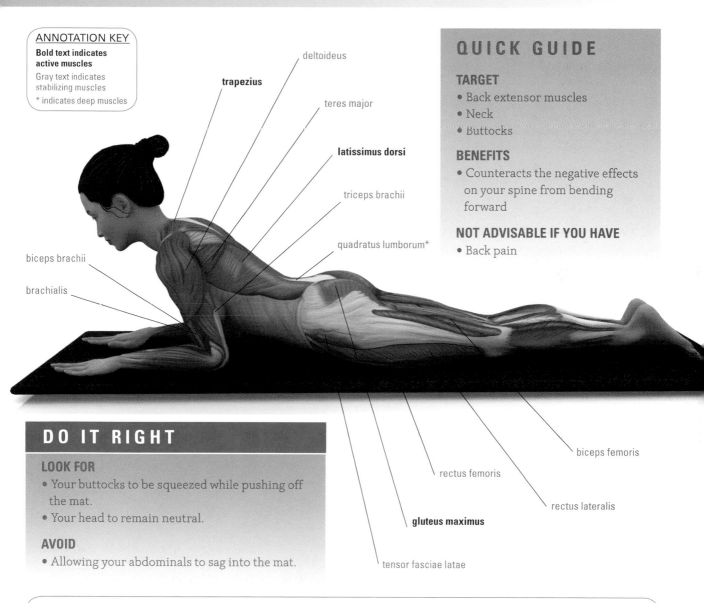

ANNOTATION KEY
**Bold text indicates
active muscles**
Gray text indicates
stabilizing muscles
* indicates deep muscles

deltoideus

trapezius

teres major

latissimus dorsi

triceps brachii

quadratus lumborum*

biceps brachii

brachialis

biceps femoris

rectus femoris

rectus lateralis

gluteus maximus

tensor fasciae latae

QUICK GUIDE

TARGET
- Back extensor muscles
- Neck
- Buttocks

BENEFITS
- Counteracts the negative effects on your spine from bending forward

NOT ADVISABLE IF YOU HAVE
- Back pain

DO IT RIGHT

LOOK FOR
- Your buttocks to be squeezed while pushing off the mat.
- Your head to remain neutral.

AVOID
- Allowing your abdominals to sag into the mat.

MODIFICATIONS

More Difficult: Push further through your hands until your elbows are extended. Keep scooping your stomach in while your hips rise off the mat.

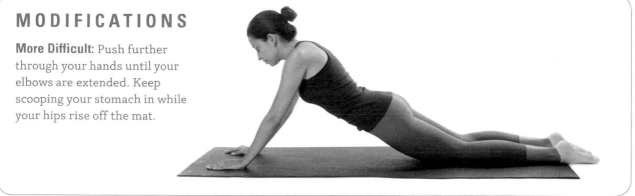

CHILD'S POSE

BEGINNER

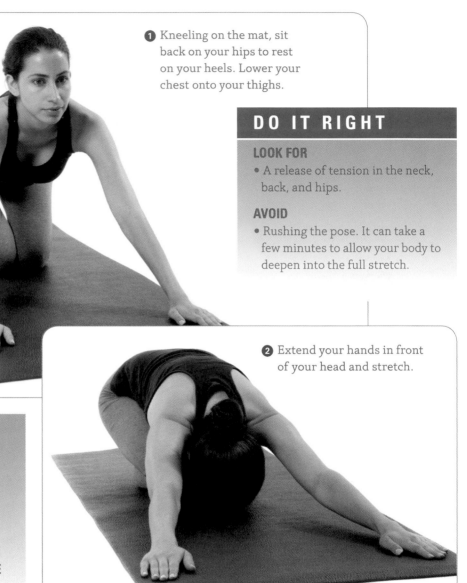

❶ Kneeling on the mat, sit back on your hips to rest on your heels. Lower your chest onto your thighs.

DO IT RIGHT

LOOK FOR
• A release of tension in the neck, back, and hips.

AVOID
• Rushing the pose. It can take a few minutes to allow your body to deepen into the full stretch.

❷ Extend your hands in front of your head and stretch.

QUICK GUIDE

TARGET
• Lower back

BENEFITS
• Stretches and relaxes the back

NOT ADVISABLE IF YOU HAVE
• Knee injury

The Child's Pose is a relaxing stretch that can be done at any point to alleviate tension in the back and hips created during your workout.

BEST FOR

• latissimus dorsi
• trapezius
• quadratus lumborum
• deltoideus
• rhomboideus
• teres major
• serratus anterior
• gluteus maximus
• erector spinae

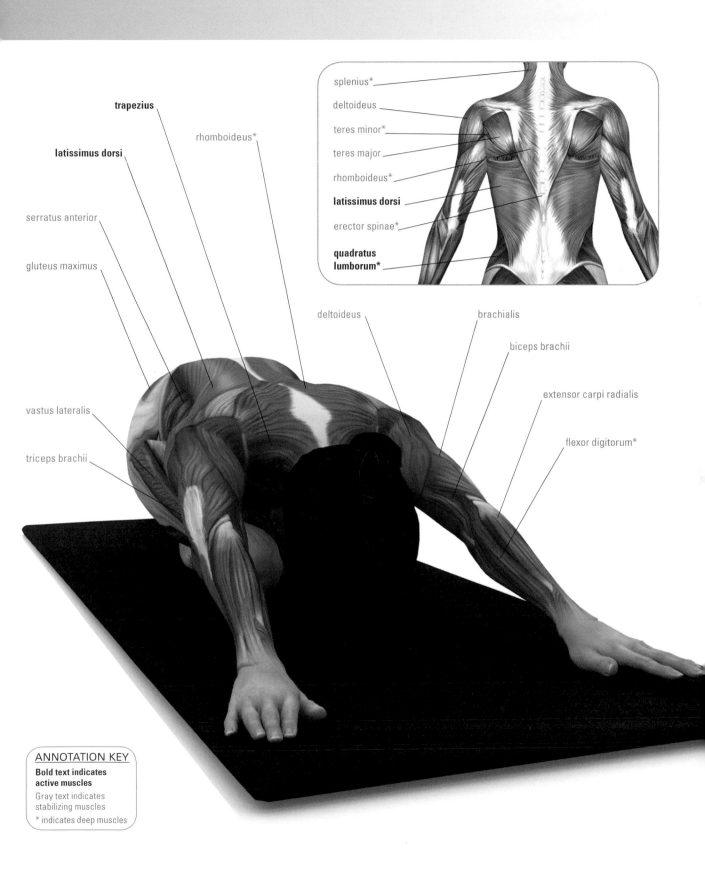

splenius*
deltoideus
teres minor*
teres major
rhomboideus*
latissimus dorsi
erector spinae*
quadratus lumborum*

trapezius

rhomboideus*

latissimus dorsi

serratus anterior

gluteus maximus

vastus lateralis

triceps brachii

deltoideus

brachialis

biceps brachii

extensor carpi radialis

flexor digitorum*

ANNOTATION KEY
Bold text indicates active muscles
Gray text indicates stabilizing muscles
* indicates deep muscles

PLANK ROLL-DOWN

BEGINNER

Many Pilates exercises act as setups or building blocks for more advanced exercises. The Plank Roll-down strengthens the arms and abdominals, homing in on the positions you will need to master to do Push-ups. The controlled up-and-down motion also targets the leg muscles.

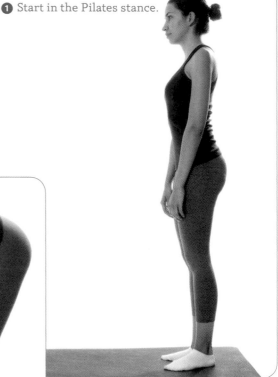

❶ Start in the Pilates stance.

❷ Bow your head and roll down, bringing your hands to the floor.

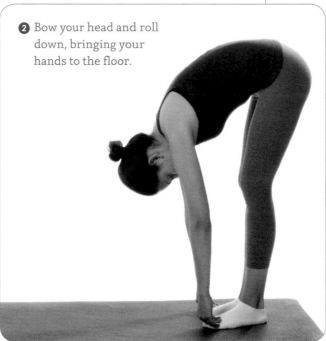

BEST FOR

- rectus abdominis
- triceps brachii
- gluteus maximus
- biceps femoris
- obliquus externus
- tensor fasciae latae
- rectus femoris
- vastus intermedius

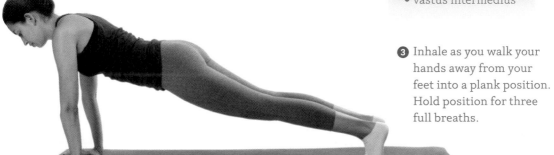

❸ Inhale as you walk your hands away from your feet into a plank position. Hold position for three full breaths.

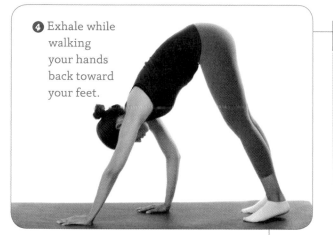

4 Exhale while walking your hands back toward your feet.

DO IT RIGHT

LOOK FOR
• Your body to be rigid when in the plank position.

AVOID
• Allowing your lower back to sag.

5 Inhale, rolling up to return to the standing Pilates stance. Repeat sequence three times.

QUICK GUIDE

TARGET
• Core muscles

BENEFITS
• Strengthens and tones abdominals, arms, and legs

NOT ADVISABLE IF YOU HAVE
• Pregnancy
• Lower-back pain

ANNOTATION KEY
Bold text indicates active muscles
Gray text indicates stabilizing muscles
* indicates deep muscles

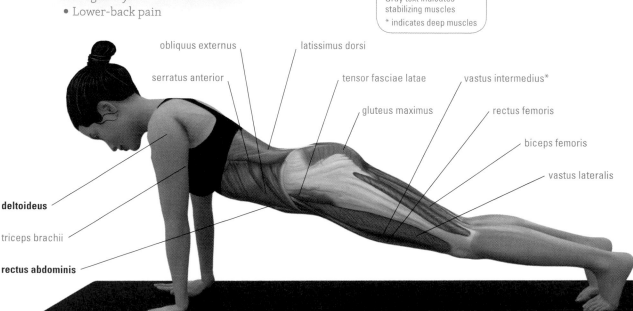

obliquus externus

latissimus dorsi

serratus anterior

tensor fasciae latae

vastus intermedius*

gluteus maximus

rectus femoris

biceps femoris

vastus lateralis

deltoideus

triceps brachii

rectus abdominis

THIGH ROCK-BACK

The Thigh Rock-back is an exercise of control, strengthening the thighs and abdominals while stretching the legs and ankles. As you practice this movement, you will be able to lean farther back, giving you a challenge even as you reach a higher skill level.

QUICK GUIDE

TARGET
- Quadriceps
- Abdominal muscles

BENEFITS
- Stretches thighs
- Increases range of motion of anterior ankle

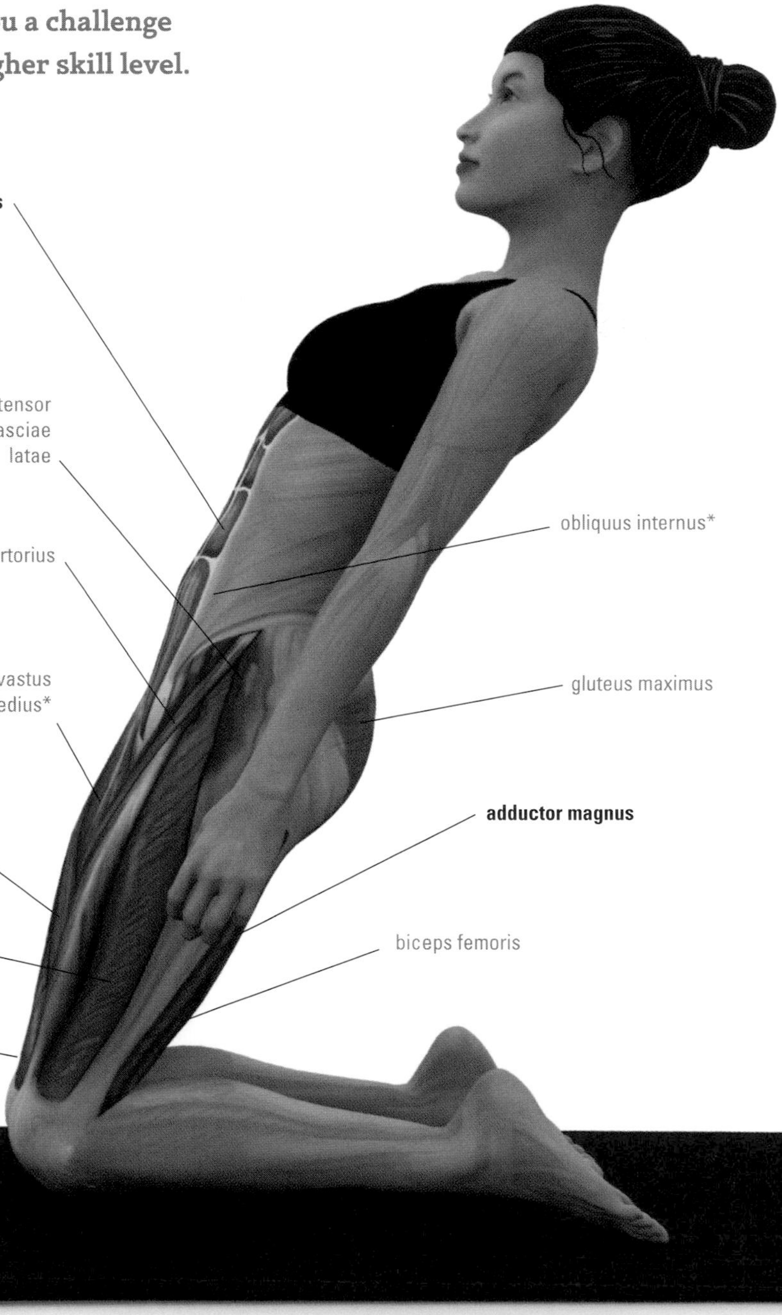

rectus abdominis

tensor fasciae latae

sartorius

vastus intermedius*

rectus femoris

vastus lateralis

vastus medialis

obliquus internus*

gluteus maximus

adductor magnus

biceps femoris

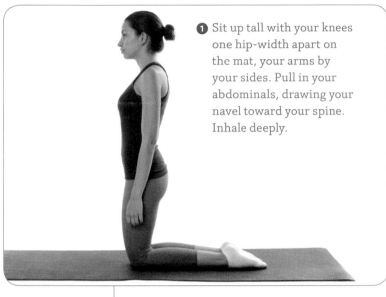

1 Sit up tall with your knees one hip-width apart on the mat, your arms by your sides. Pull in your abdominals, drawing your navel toward your spine. Inhale deeply.

DO IT RIGHT

LOOK FOR
• Creating a straight line from your torso through your knees.
• Using your abdominal muscles to maintain a controlled movement.
• Squeezing your buttock muscles.

AVOID
• Rocking so far back that you cannot return to the starting position.
• Bending in your hips.

2 Exhale and lean back, keeping your hips open and aligned with your shoulders, stretching the front of your thighs.

BEST FOR

• rectus abdominis
• rectus femoris
• vastus intermedius
• vastus medialis
• biceps femoris
• tensor fasciae latae
• gluteus maximus
• obliquus internus
• adductor magnus
• sartorius

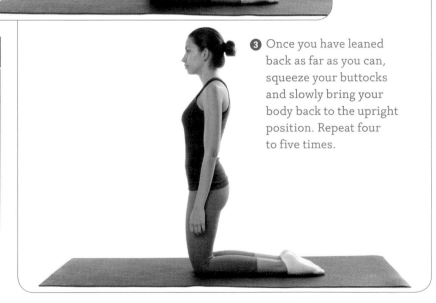

3 Once you have leaned back as far as you can, squeeze your buttocks and slowly bring your body back to the upright position. Repeat four to five times.

TENDON STRETCH

The Tendon Stretch integrates balance, coordination, resistance, and stretching to target the leg muscles. This movement also strengthens muscles in the feet.

BEST FOR

- tibialis anterior
- gastrocnemius
- soleus
- gluteus maximus
- biceps femoris
- rectus femoris
- abductor hallucis
- vastus medialis

① Standing with your feet together and parallel, extend your arms in front of your body for stability. With your feet planted firmly on the floor, curl your toes upward.

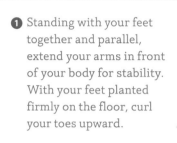

② Draw in your abdominal muscles and bend into a squat. Keep your heels planted on the floor and your chest as upright as possible, resisting the urge to bend too far forward.

QUICK GUIDE

TARGET
- Arches of feet
- Calf muscles

BENEFITS
- Lengthens and strengthens calf muscles
- Improves balance

NOT ADVISABLE IF YOU HAVE
- Foot pain

③ Exhale, returning to the original position. Imagine pressing into the floor as you rise, creating your body's own resistance in your leg muscles. Repeat five to six times.

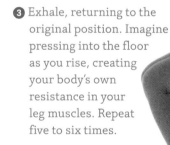

DO IT RIGHT

LOOK FOR

- Your chest to remain upright.
- Your abdominals to be pulled in toward your spine.
- Your toes to curl upward throughout the movement.

AVOID

- Allowing your heels to come off the floor.
- Rising to the standing position too quickly.

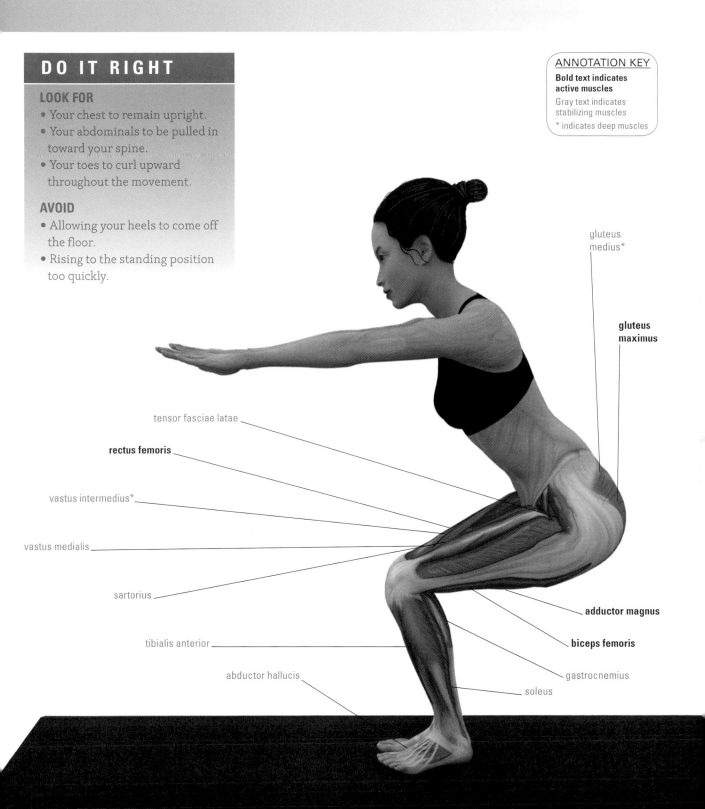

gluteus medius*

gluteus maximus

tensor fasciae latae

rectus femoris

vastus intermedius*

vastus medialis

sartorius

tibialis anterior

abductor hallucis

adductor magnus

biceps femoris

gastrocnemius

soleus

SINGLE-LEG BALANCE

BEGINNER

The Single-leg Balance is a simple movement executed in three directions: front, back, and side. Extending the leg in three directions helps improve balance and overall strength in the legs and feet.

QUICK GUIDE

TARGET
• Center balance

BENEFITS
• Improves balance
• Strengthens feet and ankles

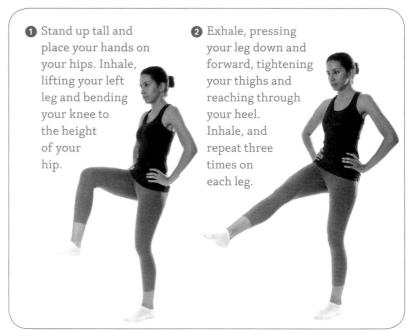

❶ Stand up tall and place your hands on your hips. Inhale, lifting your left leg and bending your knee to the height of your hip.

❷ Exhale, pressing your leg down and forward, tightening your thighs and reaching through your heel. Inhale, and repeat three times on each leg.

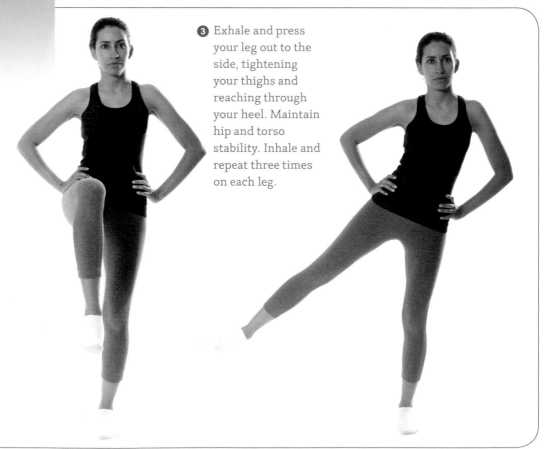

❸ Exhale and press your leg out to the side, tightening your thighs and reaching through your heel. Maintain hip and torso stability. Inhale and repeat three times on each leg.

BEST FOR

- rectus abdominis
- obliquus externus
- adductor longus
- adductor magnus
- gastrocnemius
- tibialis anterior
- biceps femoris
- tensor fasciae latae
- rectus femoris
- vastus lateralis

DO IT RIGHT

LOOK FOR

- Your spine to remain in a smooth line from neck to waist.

AVOID

- Taking your hands from your hips. If you feel yourself losing your balance, tap your lifted foot to the floor.

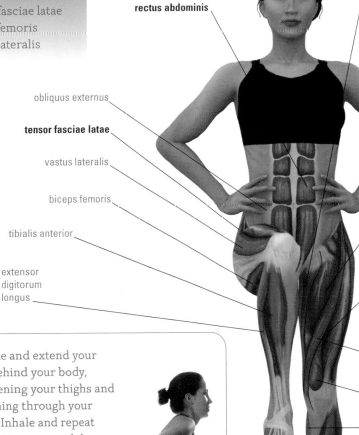

rectus abdominis
adductor magnus
obliquus externus
tensor fasciae latae
vastus lateralis
biceps femoris
tibialis anterior
extensor digitorum longus
adductor longus
rectus femoris
sartorius
vastus medialis
gastrocnemius
extensor hallucis
flexor hallucis

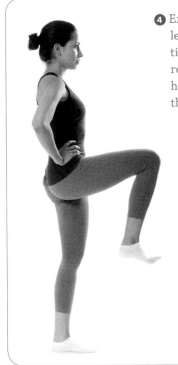
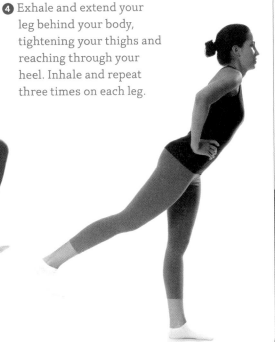

④ Exhale and extend your leg behind your body, tightening your thighs and reaching through your heel. Inhale and repeat three times on each leg.

ANNOTATION KEY

Bold text indicates active muscles

Gray text indicates stabilizing muscles

* indicates deep muscles

THE WINDMILL

BEGINNER

Stacking the spine properly is a fundamental skill to master in Pilates. The Windmill promotes spinal stacking with a slow, stretching movement.

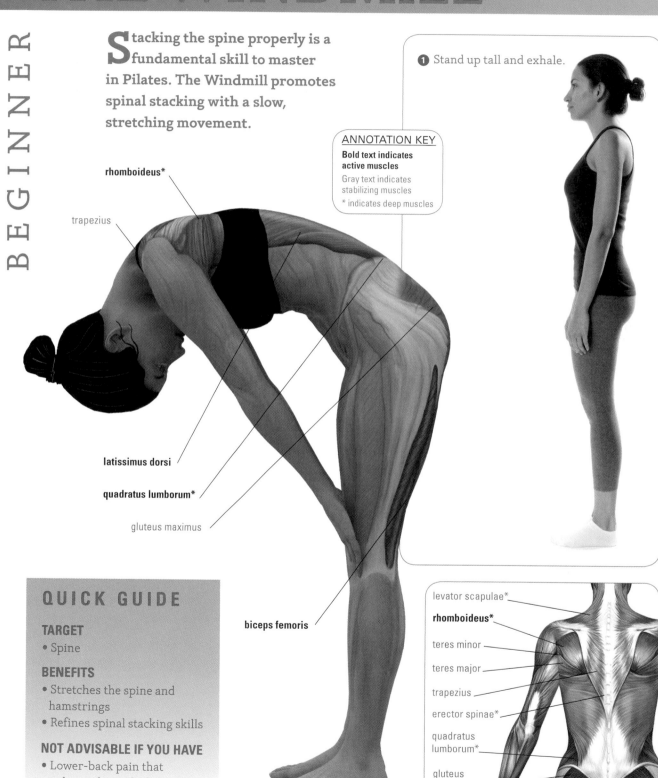

1 Stand up tall and exhale.

ANNOTATION KEY
Bold text indicates active muscles
Gray text indicates stabilizing muscles
* indicates deep muscles

rhomboideus*

trapezius

latissimus dorsi

quadratus lumborum*

gluteus maximus

biceps femoris

levator scapulae*

rhomboideus*

teres minor

teres major

trapezius

erector spinae*

quadratus lumborum*

gluteus medius*

QUICK GUIDE

TARGET
• Spine

BENEFITS
• Stretches the spine and hamstrings
• Refines spinal stacking skills

NOT ADVISABLE IF YOU HAVE
• Lower-back pain that radiates down the legs

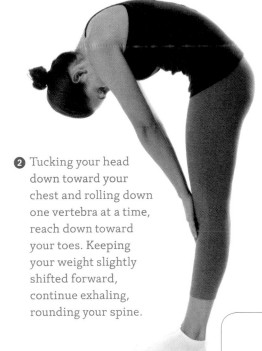

2 Tucking your head down toward your chest and rolling down one vertebra at a time, reach down toward your toes. Keeping your weight slightly shifted forward, continue exhaling, rounding your spine.

DO IT RIGHT

LOOK FOR
- Stacking your spine one vertebra at a time.
- The stretch in your back to connect with the stretch in your hamstrings.

3 When you are completely folded over, inhale and begin uncurling your spine, stacking the spine from your hips up to your shoulders. Roll your shoulders back and stand up tall. Repeat three times.

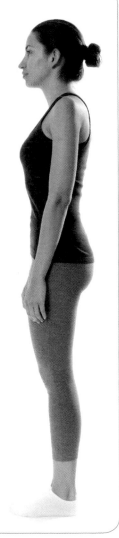

BEST FOR

- latissimus dorsi
- erector spinae
- rhomboideus
- quadratus lumborum
- biceps femoris
- gluteus maximus

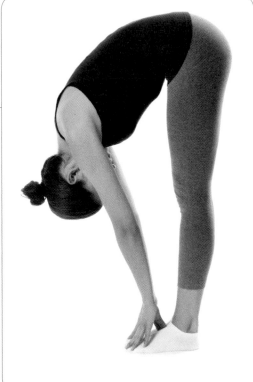

HEEL BEATS

B E G I N N E R

While the Heel Beats exercise is done lying down comfortably, it tones and strengthens the muscles all the way from the back of the neck to the tendons of the feet.

DO IT RIGHT

LOOK FOR
• Your buttocks and your abdominals to be squeezed while beating your heels.
• Your breathing to remain steady.

AVOID
• Tensing your shoulders.

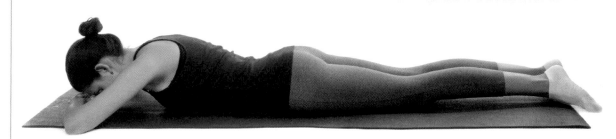

❶ Lie facedown with your hands underneath your forehead, palms down. Draw your shoulders down away from your ears. Turn your legs out from the top of your hips and pull your inner thighs together.

QUICK GUIDE

TARGET
• Core

BENEFITS
• Encourages muscles from the entire body to work together
• Lengthens extension muscles

NOT ADVISABLE IF YOU HAVE
• Back pain

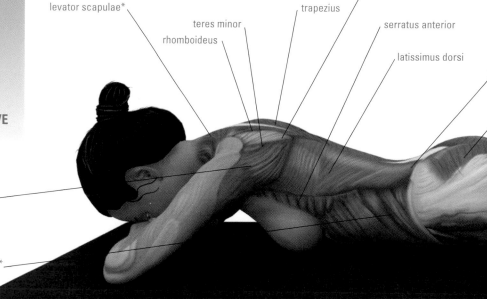

levator scapulae*

teres minor

rhomboideus

trapezius

teres major

serratus anterior

latissimus dorsi

deltoideus

transversus abdominis*

② Pull your navel off the mat and toward your spine, pressing your pubic bone into the mat. Lengthen your legs and lift them off the mat, tightening your thigh muscles.

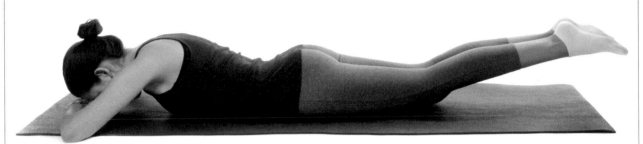

③ Press your heels together and then separate them in a rapid but controlled motion. Beat heels together for eight counts, then return to the starting position. Repeat sequence six to eight times.

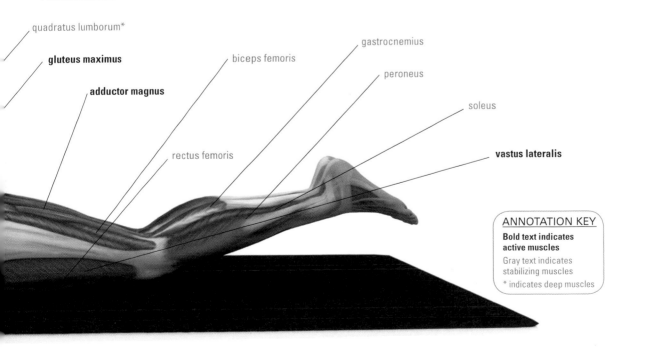

quadratus lumborum*

gluteus maximus

adductor magnus

biceps femoris

gastrocnemius

peroneus

soleus

rectus femoris

vastus lateralis

ANNOTATION KEY
Bold text indicates active muscles
Gray text indicates stabilizing muscles
* indicates deep muscles

SAMPLE SEQUENCES

BEGINNER

The following sample sequences provide you with a comprehensive total-body workout, using the exercises that you have learned in this chapter. These exercises are the basis for more advanced exercises that you will learn as you progress through this book. Two routines are provided to guide you through a mastery of the beginner level. There are numerous ways in which this exercise program can be configured. These two routines were created to provide you with the best means to activate and

LEARNING AND PERFECTING THE BASICS I

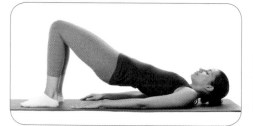

Single-leg Balance

Tendon Stretch

The Windmill

Thigh Rock-back

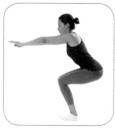

Child's Pose

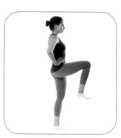

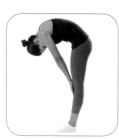

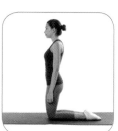

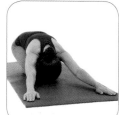

Rolling Like a Ball

Spine Stretch II

Spine Twist

Roll-down

Half Curl

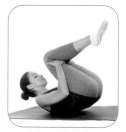

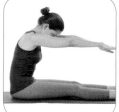

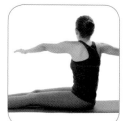

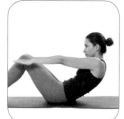

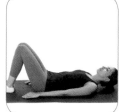

Bridge I

Single-leg Circles

Tiny Steps

Child's Pose

STRETCHES

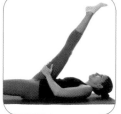

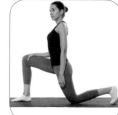

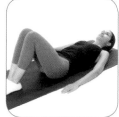

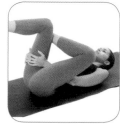

Hamstring Stretch

Hip Flexor Stretch

Lumbar Stretch

Piriformis Stretch

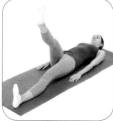

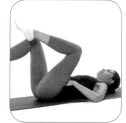

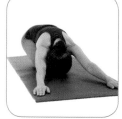

strengthen key muscles of the core and to target related muscles that will be used in synergy with one another throughout the book. You can alter the order of these exercises as you wish, and you should perform each exercise four to six times.

In the first section of this book, stretching exercises are provided to give you overall flexibility and to keep your muscles lengthened. Performing these exercises before each workout will loosen your muscles and prepare you for your workout.

LEARNING AND PERFECTING THE BASICS II

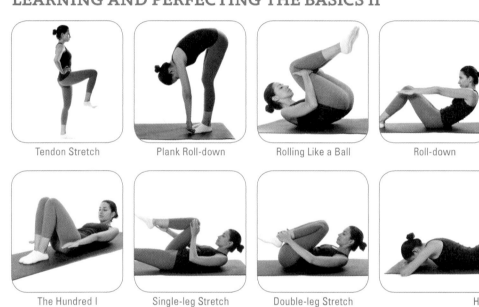

Tendon Stretch

Plank Roll-down

Rolling Like a Ball

Roll-down

Half Curl

The Hundred I

Single-leg Stretch

Double-leg Stretch

Heel Beats

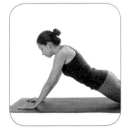

The Rising Swan

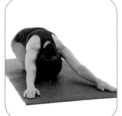

Child's Pose

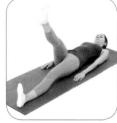

Single-leg Circles

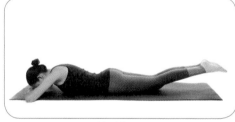

Single Leg Lift Prep

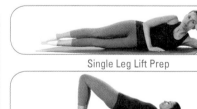

Bridge I

STRETCHES

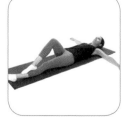

Spine Stretch

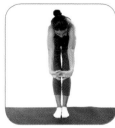

Latissimus Dorsi Stretch

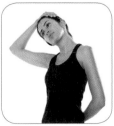

Side-bend Stretch

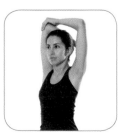

Triceps Stretch

PLANK WITH LEG LIFT

INTERMEDIATE

Connecting the legs and arms with the core, while focusing on balance and stability, is one of the most important elements of Pilates. The Plank with Leg Lift exercise helps tone all of these muscles along the body's central axis through one powerful, extending movement.

BEST FOR

- gluteus maximus
- biceps femoris
- gluteus medius
- deltoideus
- rectus femoris
- adductor magnus
- tensor fasciae latae
- rectus abdominis
- transversus abdominis
- obliquus internus
- adductor longus

QUICK GUIDE

TARGET
- Core stability
- Pelvic stabilizers
- Hip extensor muscles
- Oblique muscles

NOT ADVISABLE IF YOU HAVE
- Lower-back pain
- Wrist pain
- Knee pain while kneeling
- Inability to stabilize the spine while moving limbs

❶ Kneeling on all fours, connect with your abdominals by drawing your belly button up toward your spine in one inhalation.

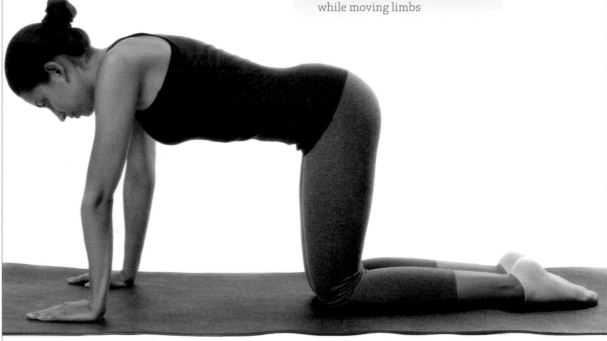

2 Exhale, slowly raising one arm and extending the opposite leg, all while keeping your torso still. Extend your arm and leg until they are both parallel to the floor, creating one long line with your body. Do not allow your pelvis to bend or rotate.

3 Inhale, bringing your arm and leg back into the starting position.

4 Exhale and repeat sequence on the other side, alternating sides six times.

DO IT RIGHT

LOOK FOR
- Maintaining a slow pace in the movement to decrease pelvic movement.

AVOID
- Tilting your pelvis during the movement—slide your leg along the surface of the mat before lifting.
- Allowing your back to sink into an arched position.

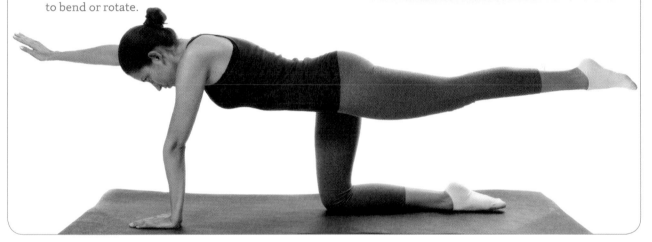

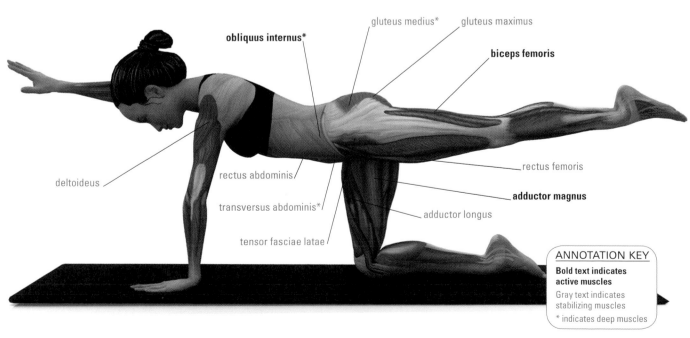

gluteus medius*
gluteus maximus
obliquus internus*
biceps femoris
deltoideus
rectus abdominis
rectus femoris
transversus abdominis*
adductor magnus
adductor longus
tensor fasciae latae

ANNOTATION KEY
Bold text indicates active muscles
Gray text indicates stabilizing muscles
* indicates deep muscles

LEG PULL-BACK

INTERMEDIATE

Similar to the Plank with Leg Lift, the Leg Pull-back targets the muscles of the legs, the abdominals, and the arm muscles. Slightly more challenging than the leg lift, this exercise demands that you maintain stability while achieving full body extension and flexion.

DO IT RIGHT

AVOID

• Allowing your shoulders to sink into their sockets. If your legs do not feel strong enough to support your body, slightly bend your knees.

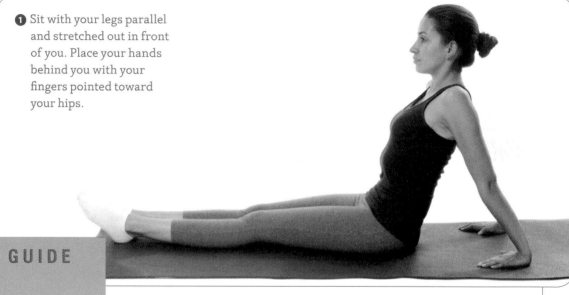

❶ Sit with your legs parallel and stretched out in front of you. Place your hands behind you with your fingers pointed toward your hips.

QUICK GUIDE

TARGET

• Hip extensor muscles
• Core stabilizers
• Arm muscles
• Leg muscles

NOT ADVISABLE IF YOU HAVE

• Wrist pain
• Shoulder injury
• Knee pain while kneeling
• Shooting pains down leg

❷ Press up through your arms and lift your chest up, squeezing your buttocks and lifting your hips while pressing your heels into the floor. Continue lifting your pelvis until your body forms a long line from your shoulders to your feet.

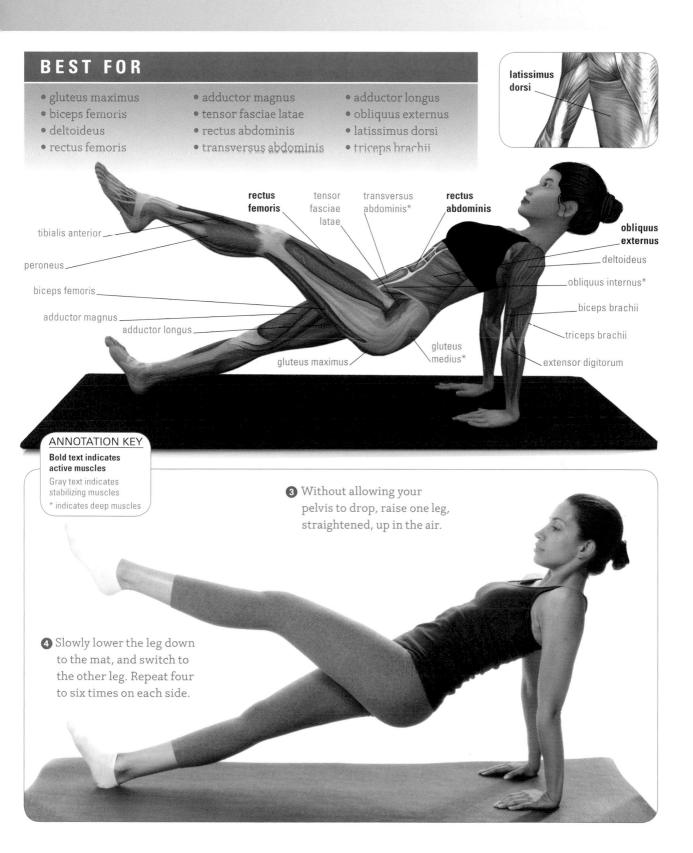

BEST FOR

- gluteus maximus
- biceps femoris
- deltoideus
- rectus femoris
- adductor magnus
- tensor fasciae latae
- rectus abdominis
- transversus abdominis
- adductor longus
- obliquus externus
- latissimus dorsi
- triceps brachii

latissimus dorsi

rectus femoris

tensor fasciae latae

transversus abdominis*

rectus abdominis

obliquus externus

tibialis anterior

peroneus

biceps femoris

adductor magnus

adductor longus

gluteus maximus

gluteus medius*

deltoideus

obliquus internus*

biceps brachii

triceps brachii

extensor digitorum

ANNOTATION KEY

Bold text indicates active muscles

Gray text indicates stabilizing muscles

* indicates deep muscles

3 Without allowing your pelvis to drop, raise one leg, straightened, up in the air.

4 Slowly lower the leg down to the mat, and switch to the other leg. Repeat four to six times on each side.

THE SEAL

INTERMEDIATE

The Seal is a fun way to target the core muscles while enjoying a back massage. Rolling out the back feels good, and finding your body's balance point at the top of the roll engages your pelvic stabilizers. While doing this exercise, make sure that you are not relying on your momentum to roll. This exercise is all about control.

DO IT RIGHT

LOOK FOR
• Allowing your momentum to help you roll backward.

AVOID
• Allowing your back to make a "thumping" sound; this indicates that you need to draw in the abdominal muscles to create a smooth, fluid movement.
• Rolling too far back on your neck. Roll only as far as your shoulder blades.

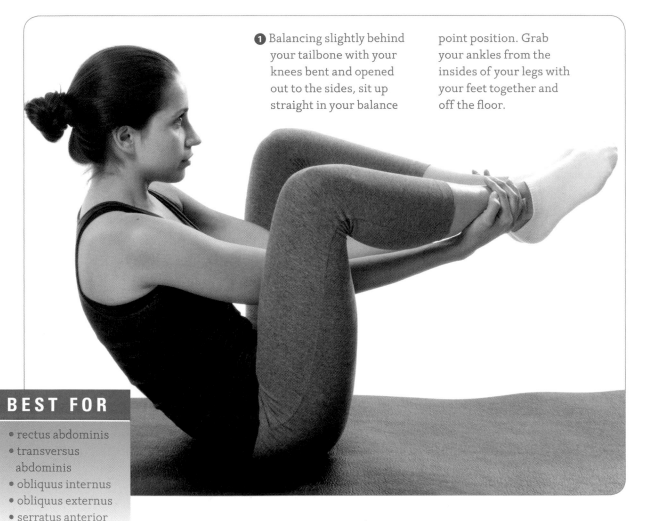

❶ Balancing slightly behind your tailbone with your knees bent and opened out to the sides, sit up straight in your balance point position. Grab your ankles from the insides of your legs with your feet together and off the floor.

BEST FOR
• rectus abdominis
• transversus abdominis
• obliquus internus
• obliquus externus
• serratus anterior

2 Inhale, rolling onto your upper back. Use your lower abdominals to scoop and lift your hips, squeezing your buttocks to give you a little extra lift.

3 Exhale, returning to your balance point. Use your abdominals to slow your momentum as you return to the starting position.

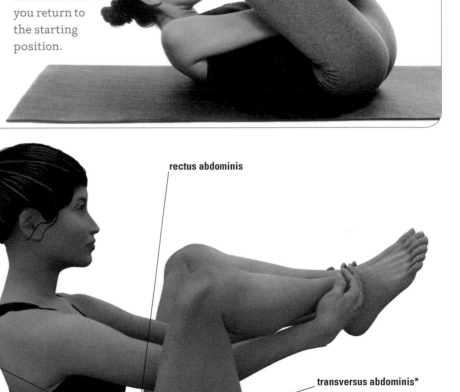

rectus abdominis

serratus anterior

obliquus externus

transversus abdominis*

obliquus internus*

ANNOTATION KEY
**Bold text indicates
active muscles**
Gray text indicates
stabilizing muscles
* indicates deep muscles

THE SAW

INTERMEDIATE

Frequently, tight back muscles and torso immobility are connected with similar issues in the legs. The Saw exercise opens up the back and hips while stretching the hamstring muscles.

BEST FOR

- biceps femoris
- rectus femoris
- obliquus internus
- rectus abdominis
- latissimus dorsi
- multifidus spinae
- quadratus lumborum
- rhomboideus

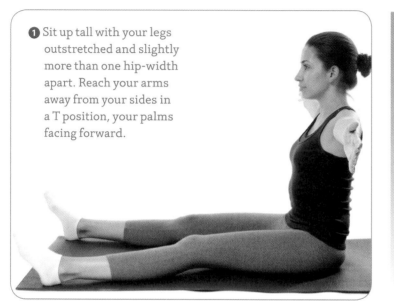

1 Sit up tall with your legs outstretched and slightly more than one hip-width apart. Reach your arms away from your sides in a T position, your palms facing forward.

QUICK GUIDE

TARGET
- Oblique muscles
- Lumbar stabilizer (multifidus spinae)

BENEFITS
- Increases mobility of the torso
- Increases the articulation of the spine

NOT ADVISABLE IF YOU HAVE
- Back pain, with pain radiating down the leg

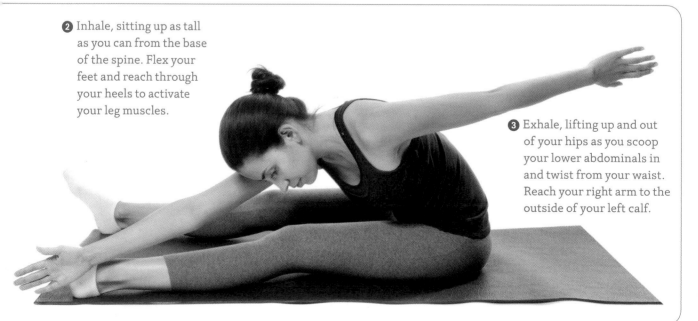

2 Inhale, sitting up as tall as you can from the base of the spine. Flex your feet and reach through your heels to activate your leg muscles.

3 Exhale, lifting up and out of your hips as you scoop your lower abdominals in and twist from your waist. Reach your right arm to the outside of your left calf.

DO IT RIGHT

LOOK FOR
- Keeping your shoulders down and relaxed.

AVOID
- Allowing your hips to raise off the mat while twisting.
- Allowing your knees to roll in as you stretch forward.

4 Inhale, drawing your navel into your spine, then exhale, reaching a bit farther with your hand along your calf, keeping your head down and your shoulders away from your ears.

5 Inhale, and return to the erect spinal position. Exhale, and begin twisting in the other direction. Repeat three times on each side.

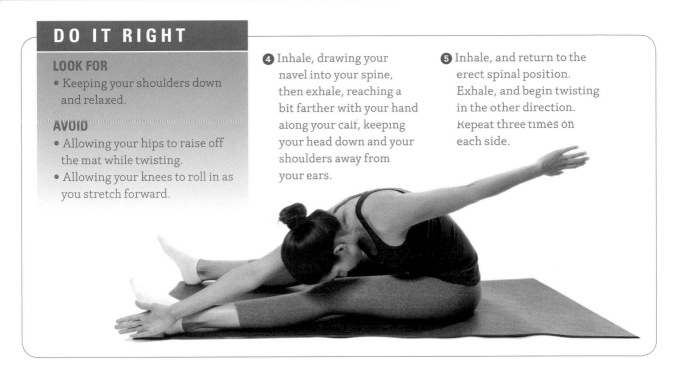

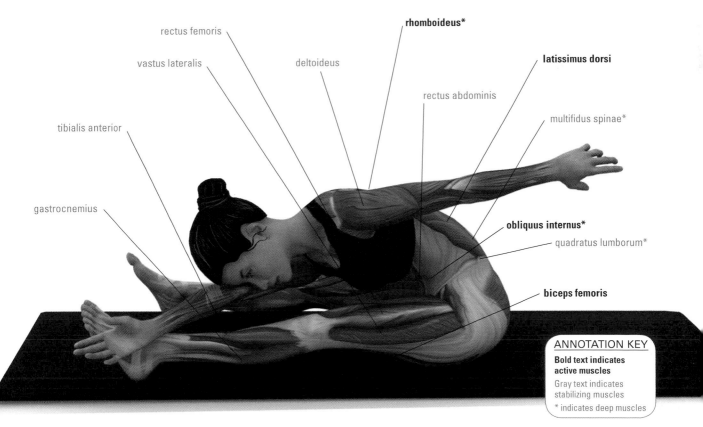

rectus femoris

vastus lateralis

deltoideus

rhomboideus*

latissimus dorsi

rectus abdominis

multifidus spinae*

tibialis anterior

gastrocnemius

obliquus internus*

quadratus lumborum*

biceps femoris

ANNOTATION KEY
Bold text indicates active muscles
Gray text indicates stabilizing muscles
* indicates deep muscles

THE CRISSCROSS

INTERMEDIATE

Exercising the oblique muscles helps to define the waist. The Crisscross exercise targets these muscles, giving you abdominals that are more toned and a back that has more rotational flexibility.

1 Bring your hands behind your head, lifting your legs in tabletop position off the floor.

DO IT RIGHT

LOOK FOR
- Drawing your stomach in as flat as possible. If you are pushing out with your stomach, you are using your back instead of your abdominal muscles.
- Keeping your elbows wide, not allowing them to fold in as you turn.
- Your twist to come from your torso.

AVOID
- Neck strain by using your hands to hold your head.
- Rocking from side to side.

QUICK GUIDE

TARGET
- Abdominal muscles

BENEFITS
- Increases stability with unilateral movement
- Increases abdominal strength and endurance

NOT ADVISABLE IF YOU HAVE
- Neck pain

BEST FOR
- rectus femoris
- vastus medialis
- sartorius
- tensor fasciae latae
- deltoideus
- rectus abdominis
- obliquus externus
- obliquus internus
- transversus abdominis

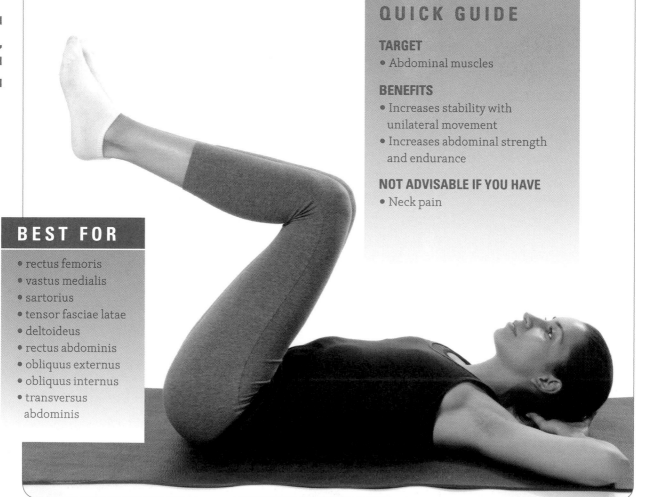

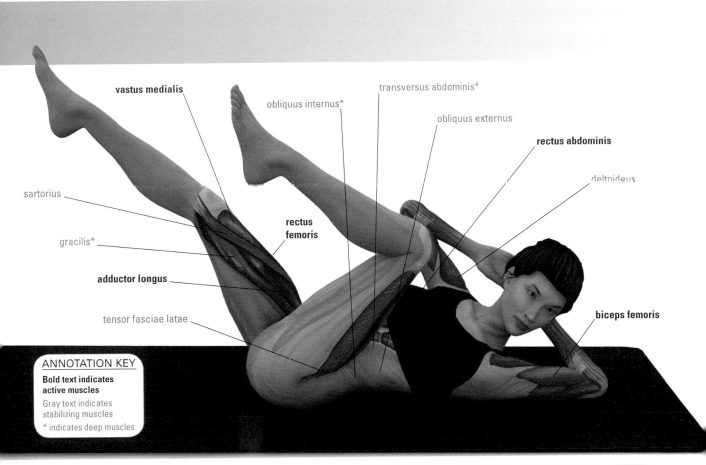

vastus medialis

obliquus internus*

transversus abdominis*

obliquus externus

rectus abdominis

deltoideus

sartorius

gracilis*

rectus femoris

adductor longus

tensor fasciae latae

biceps femoris

ANNOTATION KEY

Bold text indicates active muscles

Gray text indicates stabilizing muscles

* indicates deep muscles

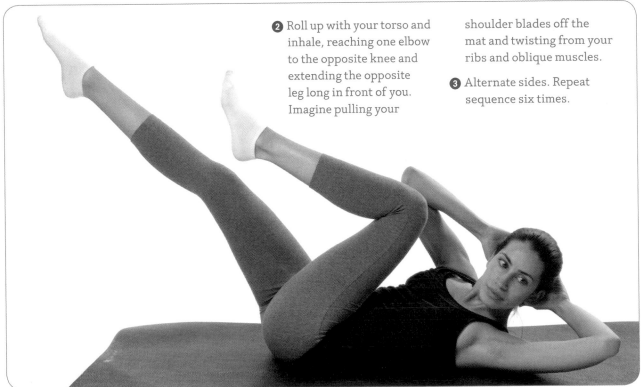

❷ Roll up with your torso and inhale, reaching one elbow to the opposite knee and extending the opposite leg long in front of you. Imagine pulling your shoulder blades off the mat and twisting from your ribs and oblique muscles.

❸ Alternate sides. Repeat sequence six times.

THE SCISSORS

INTERMEDIATE

The Scissors is one of the most popular Pilates exercises, partly because it tones and strengthens the muscles from the core through the legs. This exercise may be done almost anywhere with a small amount of floor space.

BEST FOR

- biceps femoris
- rectus femoris
- tensor fasciae latae
- rectus abdominis
- obliquus externus
- deltoideus

① Lie with your back on the mat, your arms by your sides, and your legs raised in the tabletop position. Inhale, drawing in your abdominals.

② Exhale, reaching your legs straight up and lifting your head and shoulders off the mat. Inhale, holding the position while lengthening your legs.

③ Exhale, stretching your right leg away from your body and raising your left leg toward your trunk. Hold your left leg with your hands, pulsing twice while keeping your shoulders down.

④ Inhale, switching your legs in the air, and then exhale, reaching for your opposite leg. Stabilize your pelvis and spine. Repeat sequence six to eight times on each leg.

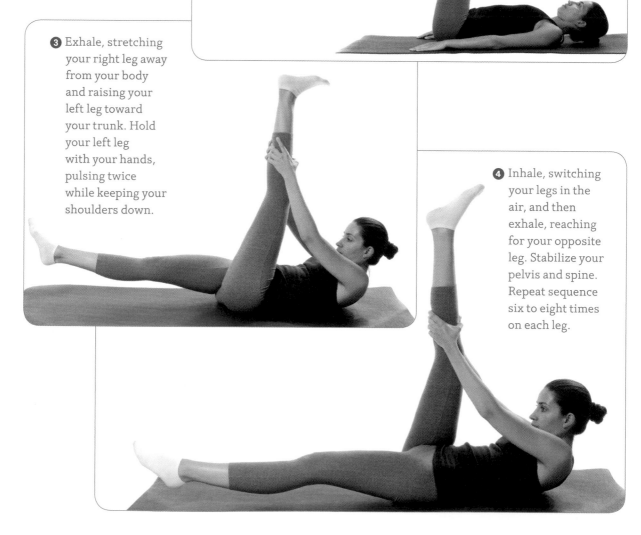

QUICK GUIDE

TARGET
• Abdominal muscles

BENEFITS
• Increases stability with unilateral movement
• Increases abdominal strength and endurance

NOT ADVISABLE IF YOU HAVE
• Tight hamstrings. If this is an issue, you may bend the knee that is moving toward your chest.

DO IT RIGHT

LOOK FOR
• Keeping your legs as straight as possible.
• Drawing your navel into your spine a little farther with each exhalation.

AVOID
• Bending your leg.

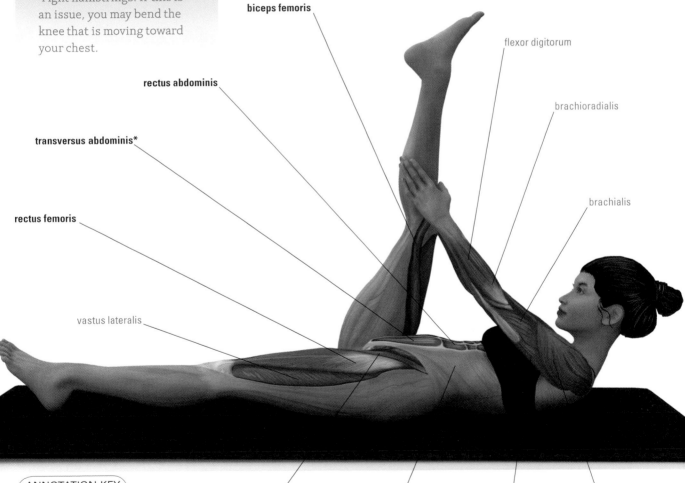

biceps femoris

flexor digitorum

brachioradialis

rectus abdominis

brachialis

transversus abdominis*

rectus femoris

vastus lateralis

ANNOTATION KEY
Bold text indicates active muscles
Gray text indicates stabilizing muscles
* indicates deep muscles

tensor fasciae latae

obliquus externus

triceps brachii

deltoideus

TEASER I

INTERMEDIATE

The Teaser I takes the Scissors exercise a step further by bringing the legs together. This means that the abdominal muscles must work to keep the legs lifted off the mat at an angle during the entire exercise. This challenge drastically improves abdominal strength.

BEST FOR

- rectus abdominis
- tensor fasciae latae
- rectus femoris
- vastus lateralis
- vastus medialis
- vastus intermedius
- adductor longus
- pectineus
- brachialis

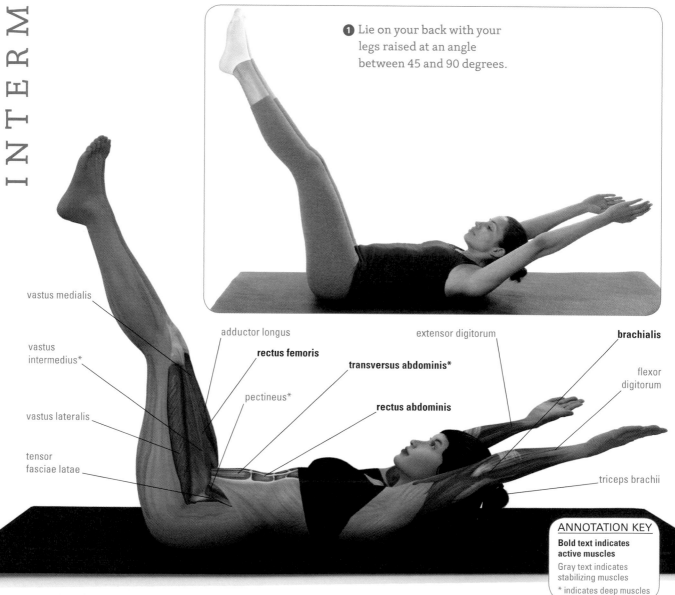

① Lie on your back with your legs raised at an angle between 45 and 90 degrees.

vastus medialis

vastus intermedius*

vastus lateralis

tensor fasciae latae

adductor longus

rectus femoris

pectineus*

transversus abdominis*

rectus abdominis

extensor digitorum

brachialis

flexor digitorum

triceps brachii

ANNOTATION KEY

Bold text indicates active muscles

Gray text indicates stabilizing muscles

* indicates deep muscles

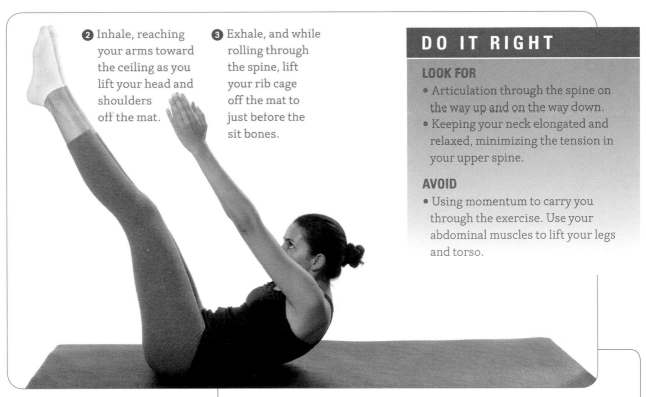

2 Inhale, reaching your arms toward the ceiling as you lift your head and shoulders off the mat.

3 Exhale, and while rolling through the spine, lift your rib cage off the mat to just before the sit bones.

DO IT RIGHT

LOOK FOR
• Articulation through the spine on the way up and on the way down.
• Keeping your neck elongated and relaxed, minimizing the tension in your upper spine.

AVOID
• Using momentum to carry you through the exercise. Use your abdominal muscles to lift your legs and torso.

QUICK GUIDE

TARGET
• Abdominal muscles

BENEFITS
• Strengthens the abdominals while mobilizing the spine

NOT ADVISABLE IF YOU HAVE
• Advanced osteoporosis
• A herniated disk
• Lower-back pain

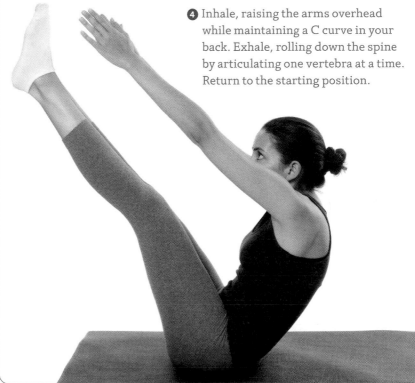

4 Inhale, raising the arms overhead while maintaining a C curve in your back. Exhale, rolling down the spine by articulating one vertebra at a time. Return to the starting position.

SIDE KICK I

INTERMEDIATE

Many people complain about the shape of their hips and thighs, looking for a way to improve muscle tone. Using the Side-kicks Prep as a foundation, the Side Kick I is a perfect exercise for targeting stubborn leg muscles. It will make your legs stronger, more flexible, and more toned.

BEST FOR

- tensor fasciae latae
- rectus femoris
- vastus lateralis
- sartorius
- adductor longus
- iliotibial band
- biceps femoris
- gluteus maximus
- gluteus medius
- vastus medialis
- vastus intermedius

❶ Lie on your side, both legs straight. Place your bottom arm underneath your head for support and the other hand in front of your torso.

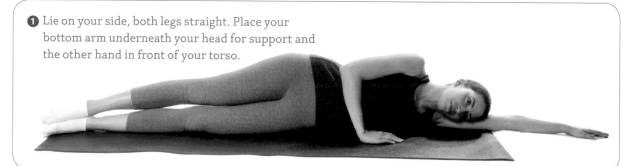

❷ Inhale, lifting your top leg to the level of your hips.

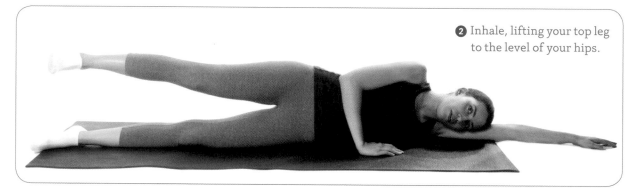

❸ Kick your leg forward, pulsing twice.

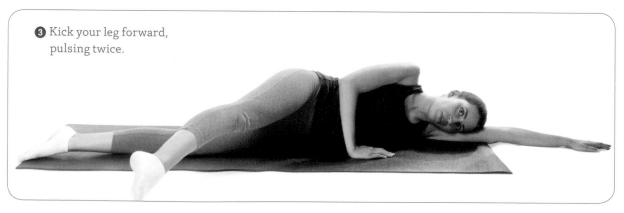

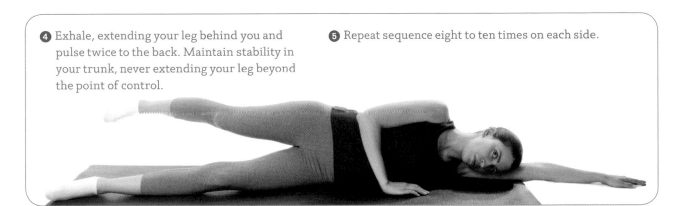

④ Exhale, extending your leg behind you and pulse twice to the back. Maintain stability in your trunk, never extending your leg beyond the point of control.

⑤ Repeat sequence eight to ten times on each side.

QUICK GUIDE

TARGET
• Hip flexor and extensor muscles

BENEFITS
• Stabilizes the spine while legs are in motion

NOT ADVISABLE IF YOU HAVE
• Shoulder injuries
• Neck injuries—if you have an injured neck, place a pillow under your head to alleviate any pain.

DO IT RIGHT

LOOK FOR
• Lengthening your legs away from your body, extending all the way through your feet.

AVOID
• Leaning on your front arm—it is just for balance. Use your core.

ANNOTATION KEY
Bold text indicates active muscles
Gray text indicates stabilizing muscles
* indicates deep muscles

gluteus maximus

gluteus medius*

tensor fasciae latae

iliotibial band

biceps femoris

vastus lateralis

vastus intermedius*

vastus medialis

sartorius

adductor longus

rectus femoris

SIDE PASSÉ

INTERMEDIATE

The Side Passé is a leg lift that tones the buttocks and outer thighs. Extending the legs elongates the muscles while strengthening them, and the core muscles work to keep the torso stable. You will feel and see the results almost immediately.

BEST FOR

- gluteus maximus
- biceps femoris
- rectus femoris
- vastus medialis
- adductor magnus
- adductor longus
- rectus abdominis
- obliquus externus
- tensor fasciae latae
- vastus lateralis

1 Lie on your side with your legs stacked in front of your body. Place your bottom hand underneath your head for support and the other hand in front of your torso.

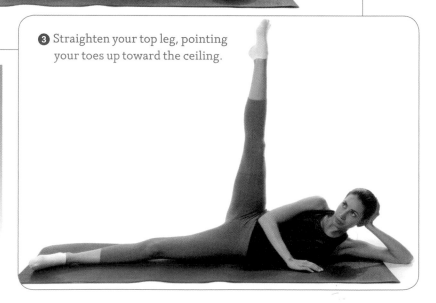

2 Inhale, bending your top leg with your knee aiming toward the ceiling. Try not to rest your foot on your bottom leg.

3 Straighten your top leg, pointing your toes up toward the ceiling.

QUICK GUIDE

BENEFITS
- Strengthens your hips, buttocks, and outer thighs

NOT ADVISABLE IF YOU HAVE
- Back pain
- Hip pain

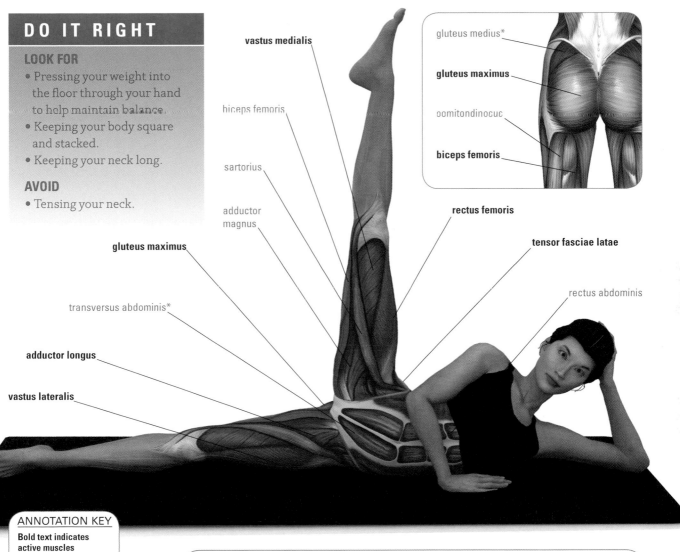

DO IT RIGHT

LOOK FOR
• Pressing your weight into the floor through your hand to help maintain balance.
• Keeping your body square and stacked.
• Keeping your neck long.

AVOID
• Tensing your neck.

vastus medialis

biceps femoris

sartorius

adductor magnus

gluteus maximus

transversus abdominis*

adductor longus

vastus lateralis

gluteus medius*

gluteus maximus

oomitondinocuc

biceps femoris

rectus femoris

tensor fasciae latae

rectus abdominis

ANNOTATION KEY
Bold text indicates active muscles
Gray text indicates stabilizing muscles
* indicates deep muscles

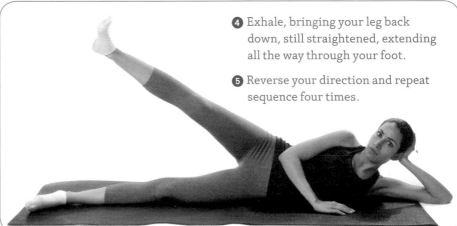

❹ Exhale, bringing your leg back down, still straightened, extending all the way through your foot.

❺ Reverse your direction and repeat sequence four times.

BICYCLE KICK

INTERMEDIATE

A variation on the Side Leg Kick, the Bicycle Kick adds a bend in the knee that mimics the bend used when riding a bicycle. Maintaining a slow, controlled movement is an important part of executing this exercise properly.

BEST FOR

- rectus abdominis
- obliquus externus
- rectus femoris
- tensor fasciae latae
- vastus lateralis
- adductor magnus
- adductor longus
- biceps femoris
- gluteus maximus

❶ Lie on your side, placing your bottom hand underneath your head for support and the other hand in front of your torso. Legs should be together and stacked in front of your body.

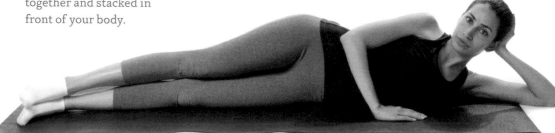

DO IT RIGHT

LOOK FOR
- Pressing your weight into the floor through your hand to help maintain balance.
- Keeping your body square and stacked.
- Keeping your neck long and relaxed.

❷ Lift your top leg up to the level of your hips. Point your foot and swing your top leg forward, extending as far as you can while still maintaining stability in your torso.

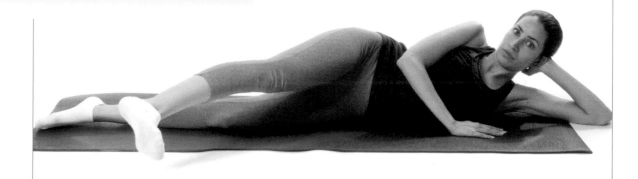

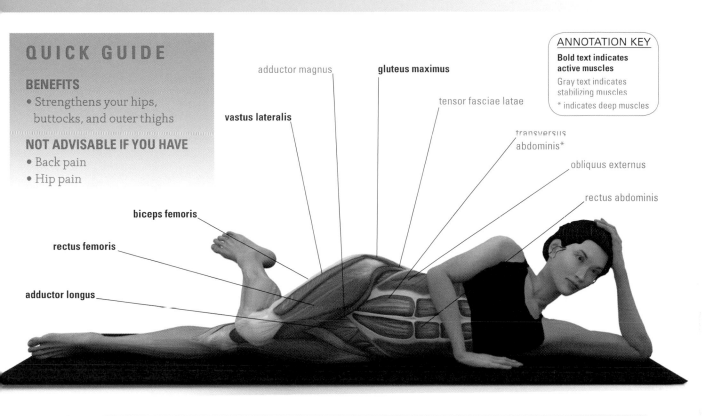

QUICK GUIDE

BENEFITS
• Strengthens your hips, buttocks, and outer thighs

NOT ADVISABLE IF YOU HAVE
• Back pain
• Hip pain

adductor magnus

gluteus maximus

tensor fasciae latae

vastus lateralis

transversus abdominis*

obliquus externus

rectus abdominis

biceps femoris

rectus femoris

adductor longus

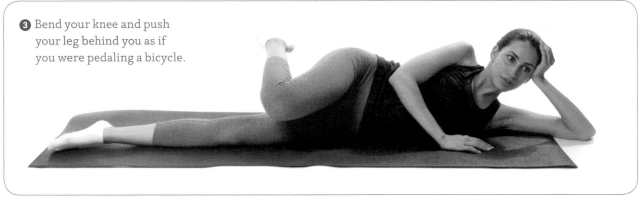

❸ Bend your knee and push your leg behind you as if you were pedaling a bicycle.

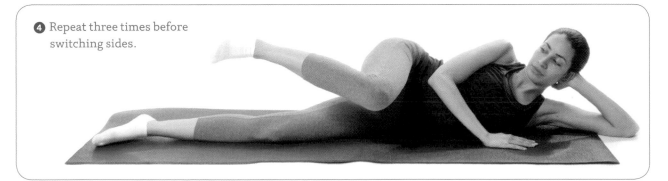

❹ Repeat three times before switching sides.

THE ROLL-UP

INTERMEDIATE

Practice control over the legs and hips while targeting the abs. The Roll-up is a classic Pilates exercise that really works the abdominal muscles, toning them far faster than even standard ab crunches.

BEST FOR

- rectus abdominis
- rectus femoris
- adductor longus
- tensor fasciae latae
- transversus abdominis
- obliquus externus

1 Lie on your back in supine position with your legs lengthened and adducted together, feet flexed.

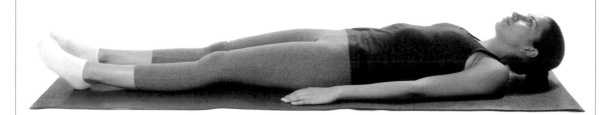

2 Inhale, reaching your arms forward while keeping your shoulders down. Exhale, gently lengthening through the back of your neck, and lift your head and shoulders. Peel your spine off the mat, pulling your navel in toward your spine.

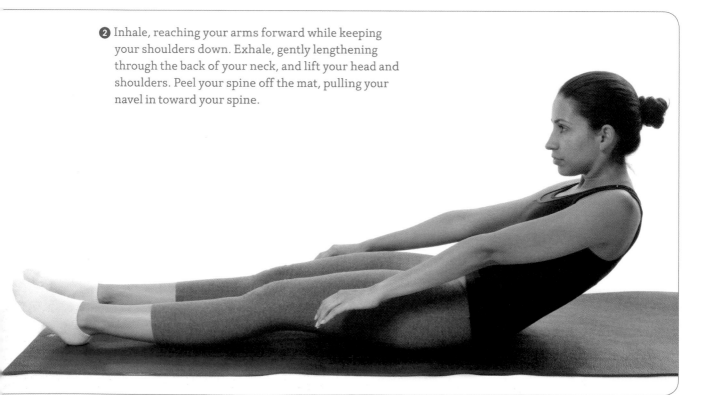

3 Exhale, curling all the way up to a sitting position, rounding the spine and lifting out of your waist.

4 Inhale and begin rolling down. Exhale, allowing the lumbar region of the spine to press into the mat first, then articulating the spine the entire way down while lengthening through the heels.

5 Repeat four to six times.

QUICK GUIDE

TARGET
• Abdominal muscles

BENEFITS
• Strengthens the abdominals while mobilizing the spine

NOT ADVISABLE IF YOU HAVE
• A herniated disk

ANNOTATION KEY
Bold text indicates active muscles
Gray text indicates stabilizing muscles
* indicates deep muscles

DO IT RIGHT

LOOK FOR
• Maintaining a slow pace in the movement to decrease pelvic movement.

AVOID
• Lifting your shoulders to help raise your torso.
• Raising your legs off the mat with the roll-up motion.

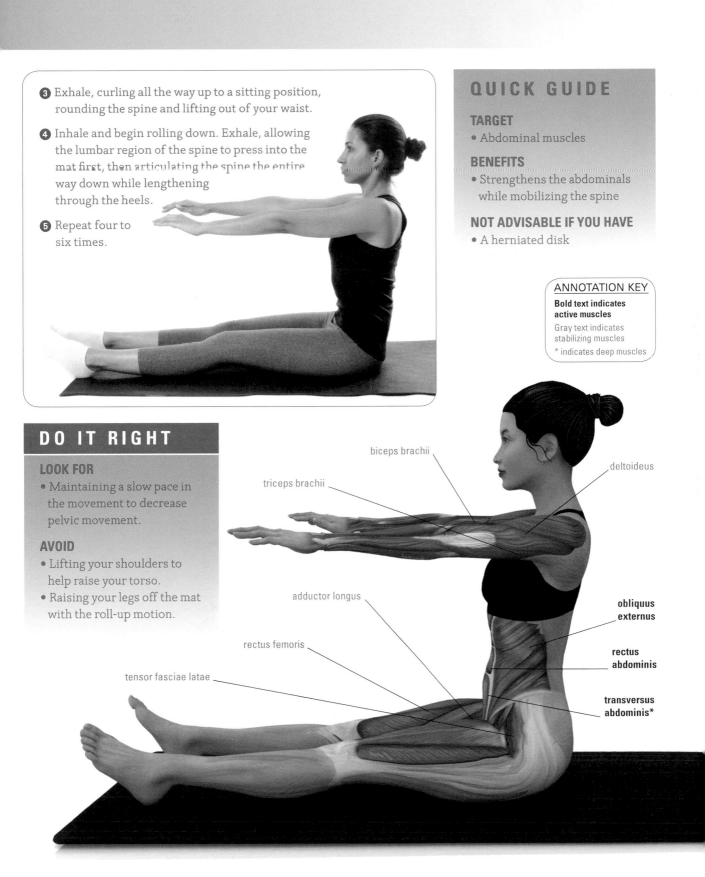

biceps brachii

triceps brachii

deltoideus

adductor longus

rectus femoris

tensor fasciae latae

obliquus externus

rectus abdominis

transversus abdominis*

SINGLE-LEG KICK

INTERMEDIATE

Use your abdominals in conjunction with your legs to build strength in your hamstrings. While performing the Single-leg Kick, your spine should remain straight, light, and as lengthened as possible.

BEST FOR

- biceps femoris
- adductor magnus
- gluteus maximus
- semimembranosus
- semitendinosus
- rectus abdominis
- obliquus externus
- transversus abdominis

❶ Lie prone on the mat with your arms flexed and elbows directly under your shoulders. Lengthen your legs and keep them adducted together.

❷ Inhale, drawing your navel in toward your spine. Exhale, bending one knee. Point your foot and pulse your bent leg eight times.

QUICK GUIDE

TARGET
- Hamstrings

BENEFITS
- Increases pelvic stability with hip extension

NOT ADVISABLE IF YOU HAVE
- Lower-back pain
- Problems with bending your knees

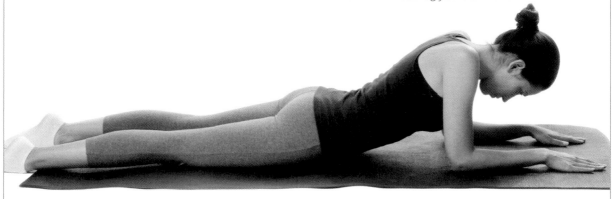

DO IT RIGHT

LOOK FOR
- Drawing in your abdominals throughout the exercise.
- Keeping the chest broad.
- Sending the tailbone toward the floor.
- Keeping your shoulders and scapula down.

AVOID
- Allowing your lower back to sag.
- Kicking too hard.

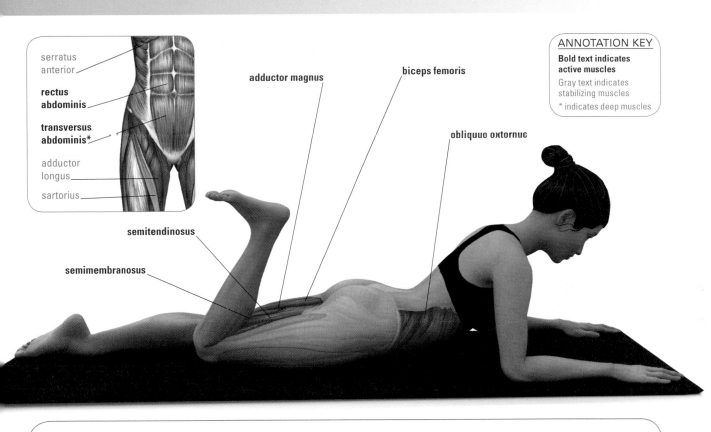

serratus anterior

rectus abdominis

transversus abdominis*

adductor longus

sartorius

semitendinosus

semimembranosus

adductor magnus

biceps femoris

obliquuo oxtornuo

❸ Exhale, then flex your foot and pulse an additional eight times.

❹ Inhale, straightening your bent leg on the mat next to the other leg. Exhale, bending your opposite leg, and repeat.

❺ Repeat the entire sequence six to eight times.

PLANK PRESS-UP

INTERMEDIATE

The Plank Press-up provides an intense workout for the arms and shoulders. In this exercise, you must depend on balance and control to avoid overextending the shoulders. Proceed at an even pace so that your shoulders stay open and don't collapse suddenly.

BEST FOR

- deltoideus
- rhomboideus
- rectus abdominis
- biceps brachii
- triceps brachii
- tensor fasciae latae
- rectus femoris
- transversus abdominis
- obliquus internus
- serratus anterior
- tibialis anterior

❶ Lying on the mat with your forearms underneath your chest, press your body up into a plank position, lengthening through your heels.

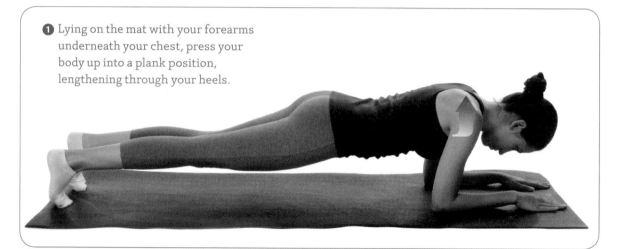

DO IT RIGHT

LOOK FOR
- Lengthening through your neck.

AVOID
- Allowing your back to sag.
- Allowing your shoulders to collapse into your shoulder joints.

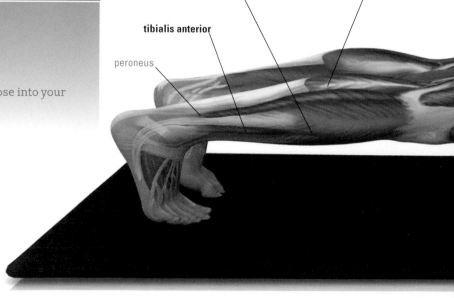

gastrocnemius

soleus

tibialis anterior

peroneus

QUICK GUIDE

TARGET
• Scapular stabilizers
• Core stability

NOT ADVISABLE IF YOU HAVE
• Shoulder injury
• Intense back pain

2 Push through your forearms to bring your shoulders up toward the ceiling. With control, lower your shoulders until you feel them coming together in your back.

3 Repeat five times.

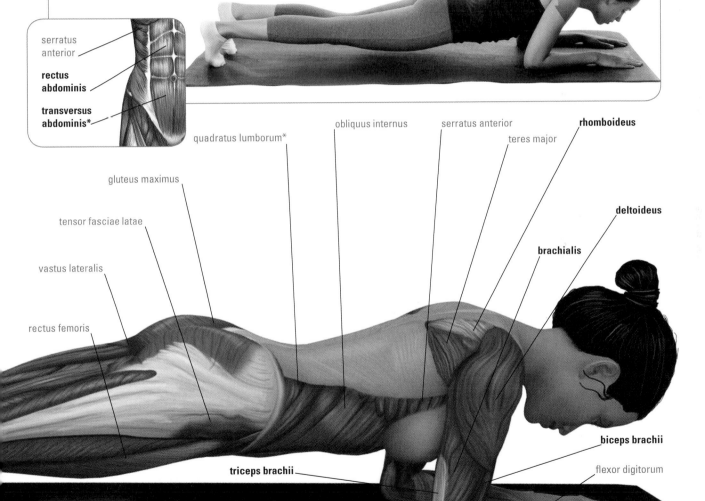

serratus anterior
rectus abdominis
transversus abdominis*

quadratus lumborum*

obliquus internus

serratus anterior

teres major

rhomboideus

gluteus maximus

tensor fasciae latae

vastus lateralis

rectus femoris

brachialis

deltoideus

triceps brachii

biceps brachii

flexor digitorum

ANNOTATION KEY
Bold text indicates active muscles
Gray text indicates stabilizing muscles
* indicates deep muscles

ROLLOVER/HIP UP

INTERMEDIATE

Practice control over the legs and hips while targeting the abdominals. The Rollover/Hip Up stretches the back and hamstrings and works the abdominals at the same time. The head and upper vertebrae should remain stable on the mat, allowing you to precisely articulate up and down the spine.

BEST FOR

- biceps femoris
- rectus femoris
- rectus abdominis
- transversus abdominis
- obliquus externus
- obliquus internus
- deltoideus

❶ Lie in supine position on the mat with your arms alongside your body.

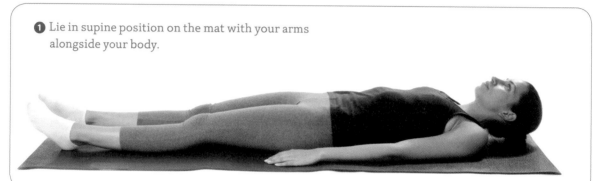

QUICK GUIDE

TARGET
- Abdominals

BENEFITS
- Strengthens the abdominals to lift the lower body and mobilize the spine

NOT ADVISABLE IF YOU HAVE
- Cervical issues
- A herniated disk

❷ Inhale, raising your legs perpendicular to the floor.

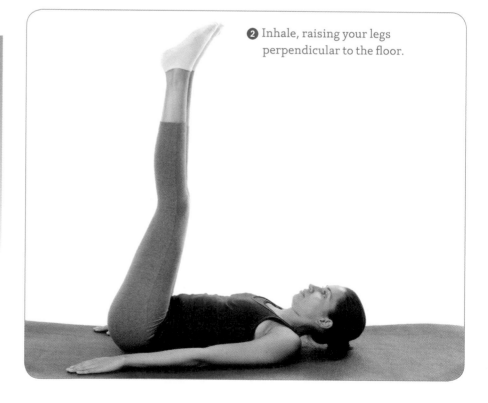

DO IT RIGHT

LOOK FOR
- Pressing your arms into the mat for extra power.
- If you have difficulty with keeping your legs pressed together, cross your legs before squeezing them together.

AVOID
- Lifting your head off the mat.
- Flopping, rather than rolling over.

❸ Exhale, drawing your legs back toward your head. Roll your lower back and rib cage off the mat, extending your legs until they are parallel to the floor.

❹ Inhale, raise the legs to hip level, and exhale as you lower the spine, articulating one vertebra at a time back to the starting position. Repeat sequence four to six times.

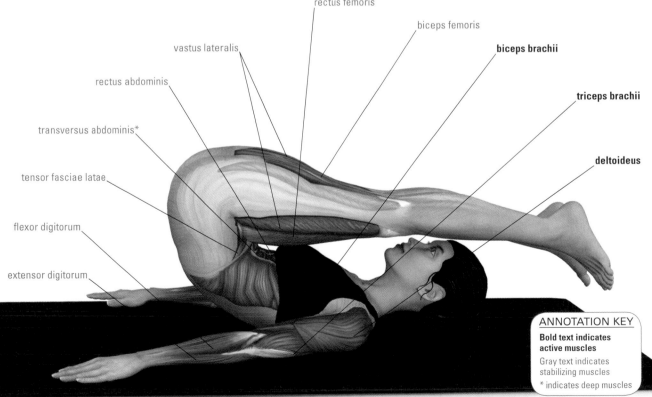

rectus femoris

biceps femoris

biceps brachii

vastus lateralis

rectus abdominis

triceps brachii

transversus abdominis*

tensor fasciae latae

deltoideus

flexor digitorum

extensor digitorum

ANNOTATION KEY
Bold text indicates active muscles
Gray text indicates stabilizing muscles
* indicates deep muscles

THE MERMAID

INTERMEDIATE

Focusing on the chest and back, the Mermaid sets the stage for a complete stretch, engaging much of the upper body. This exercise lengthens and strengthens the lateral obliques, the muscles that shape the waistline, helping to eliminate the excess bulges around the sides, known as "love handles," and any "spare tire" around the midsection. Make sure to find a comfortable position before starting so that your torso is free to move.

BEST FOR

- rectus abdominis
- transversus abdominis
- obliquus internus
- obliquus externus
- latissimus dorsi

❶ Sit to one side with your knees bent and your legs folded one on top of the other. Place your hand on your ankles. Inhale, reaching your other arm toward the ceiling.

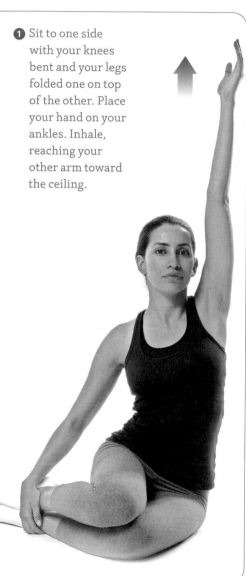

❷ Exhale, reaching your arm in the direction of your ankles, pulling your navel into your spine and rotating the torso slightly backward.

❸ Inhale, returning to the starting position. Repeat on the other side.

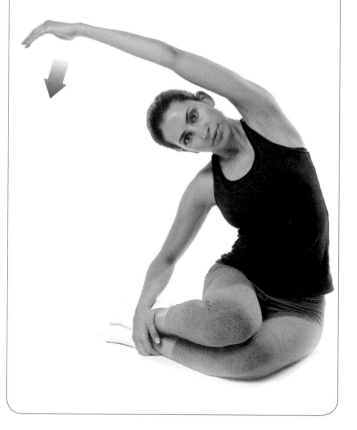

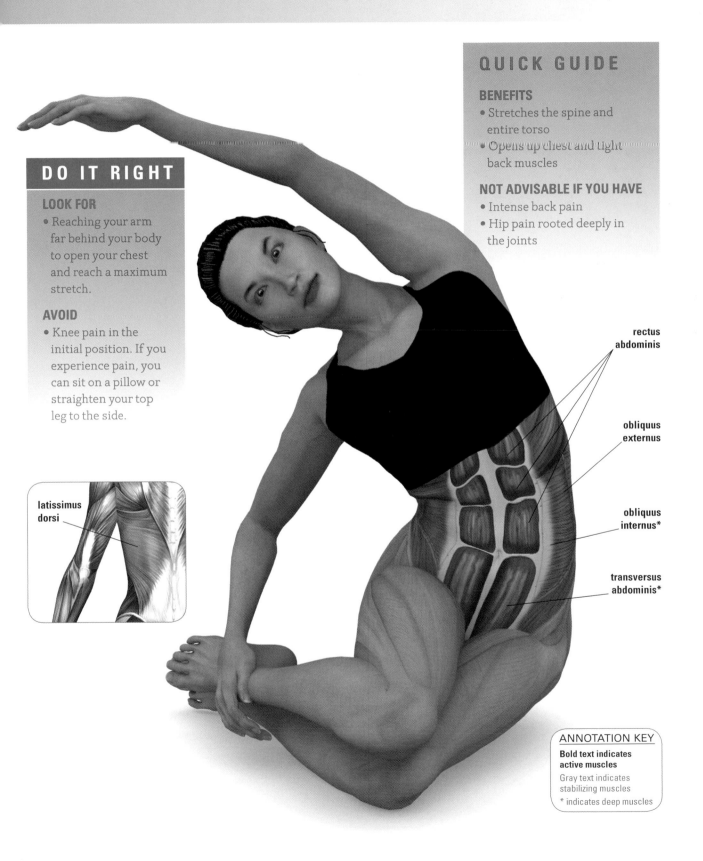

QUICK GUIDE

BENEFITS
- Stretches the spine and entire torso
- Opens up chest and tight back muscles

NOT ADVISABLE IF YOU HAVE
- Intense back pain
- Hip pain rooted deeply in the joints

DO IT RIGHT

LOOK FOR
- Reaching your arm far behind your body to open your chest and reach a maximum stretch.

AVOID
- Knee pain in the initial position. If you experience pain, you can sit on a pillow or straighten your top leg to the side.

rectus abdominis

obliquus externus

obliquus internus*

transversus abdominis*

latissimus dorsi

ANNOTATION KEY

Bold text indicates active muscles

Gray text indicates stabilizing muscles

* indicates deep muscles

SWIMMING

In this fun exercise, you can engage the same muscles that you use while swimming—which is just about every part of the body—without stepping into the pool. Using the mat for stability, aim for a long, full stretch in the arms and legs. As your head and shoulders come up off the mat, let your spine lengthen as well.

BEST FOR

- gluteus maximus
- biceps femoris
- quadratus lumborum
- rhomboideus
- latissimus dorsi
- erector spinae

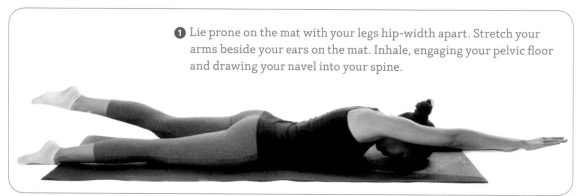

❶ Lie prone on the mat with your legs hip-width apart. Stretch your arms beside your ears on the mat. Inhale, engaging your pelvic floor and drawing your navel into your spine.

❷ Exhale, extending through your upper back as you lift your right arm and left leg simultaneously. Lift your head and shoulders off the mat.

❸ Inhale, lowering your arm and leg to the starting position, maintaining a stretch in your limbs throughout.

QUICK GUIDE

TARGET
- Spinal extensor
- Hip extensors

BENEFITS
- Strengthens hip and spine extensors
- Challenges stabilization of the spine against rotation

NOT ADVISABLE IF YOU HAVE
- Lower-back pain
- Extreme kyphosis
- Lordosis of the spine

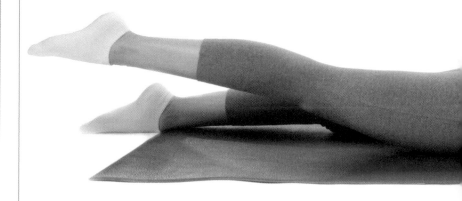

DO IT RIGHT

LOOK FOR
- Extending your limbs as long as possible in opposite directions.
- Squeezing your buttocks and drawing your navel into your spine throughout the exercise.
- Lengthening and relaxing your neck.

AVOID
- Raising your shoulders up to your ears.

> ### ANNOTATION KEY
> **Bold text indicates active muscles**
> Gray text indicates stabilizing muscles
> * indicates deep muscles

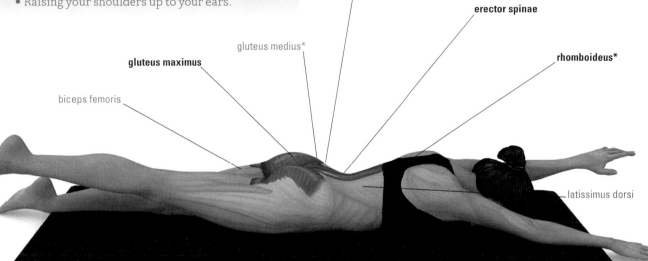

quadratus lumborum

erector spinae

rhomboideus*

gluteus medius*

gluteus maximus

biceps femoris

latissimus dorsi

4 Exhale, extending your opposite arm and leg off the floor, lengthening and lifting your head and shoulders off the mat.

5 Inhale, elongating your limbs as you return to the starting position. Repeat six to eight times.

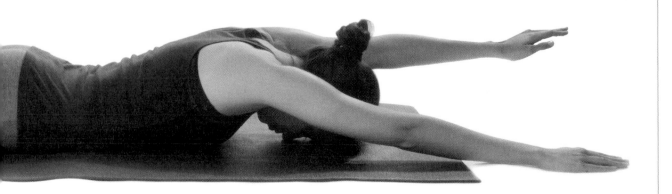

SIDE BEND I

INTERMEDIATE

The Side Bend I is a classic Pilates exercise that works to strengthen your core and increase spine flexibility. By maintaining a straight and even spine through the hips, you will transfer weight from the arms and upper body, avoiding unnecessary strain. Your shoulders are particularly vulnerable in this exercise—keep them supported and stable.

DO IT RIGHT

LOOK FOR
- Lifting your hips up high to take some weight off your upper body.
- Elongating your limbs as much as possible.

AVOID
- Allowing your shoulders to sink into their sockets or rise up to your ears.

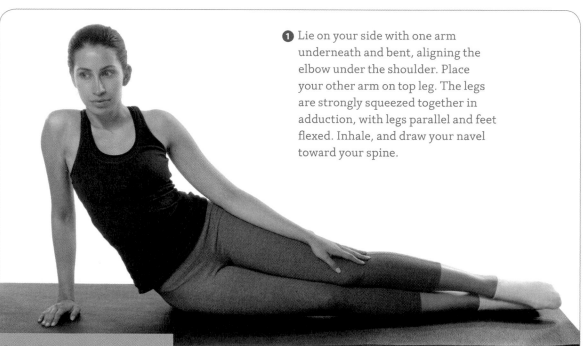

① Lie on your side with one arm underneath and bent, aligning the elbow under the shoulder. Place your other arm on top leg. The legs are strongly squeezed together in adduction, with legs parallel and feet flexed. Inhale, and draw your navel toward your spine.

QUICK GUIDE

TARGET
- Leg abductors and adductors
- Latissimus dorsi
- Pectoralis muscles

BENEFITS
- Stabilizes the spine in neutral with the support of the shoulder girdle

NOT ADVISABLE IF YOU HAVE
- Rotator cuff injury
- Neck issues

BEST FOR

- adductor magnus
- latissimus dorsi
- pectoralis minor
- pectoralis major
- triceps brachii
- obliquus externus
- obliquus internus
- gluteus medius

② Exhale, press into the elbow, and lift the hips off the mat, creating a straight line between the heels and the head. Inhale, slowly returning to the starting position. Repeat sequence five to six times, keeping your legs tight and buttocks squeezed.

ANNOTATION KEY
Bold text indicates active muscles
Gray text indicates stabilizing muscles
* indicates deep muscles

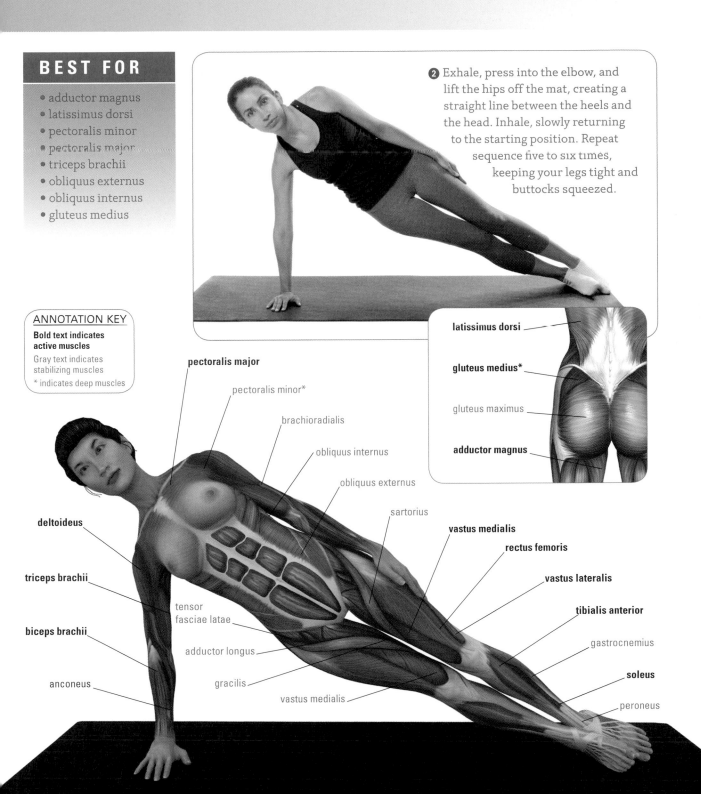

pectoralis major

pectoralis minor*

brachioradialis

obliquus internus

obliquus externus

sartorius

deltoideus

triceps brachii

biceps brachii

anconeus

tensor fasciae latae

adductor longus

gracilis

vastus medialis

vastus medialis

rectus femoris

vastus lateralis

tibialis anterior

gastrocnemius

soleus

peroneus

latissimus dorsi

gluteus medius*

gluteus maximus

adductor magnus

BRIDGE II

The Bridge II is another classic Pilates exercise that effectively strengthens the abdominal muscles and the hamstrings. To achieve the bridge position, your back and torso should do much of the work. Stability in the hips is key, also, to allow for total flexibility in the legs.

BEST FOR

- gluteus medius
- gluteus maximus
- rectus abdominis
- transversus abdominis
- quadratus lumborum
- semitendinosus
- semimembranosus
- biceps femoris
- iliopsoas
- rectus femoris
- sartorius
- tensor fasciae latae
- pectineus
- adductor longus
- adductor brevis
- gracilis

DO IT RIGHT

LOOK FOR

- Maintaining stability in your hips and torso throughout the exercise. If needed, prop yourself up with your hands beneath your hips once you are in the bridge position.
- Keeping your belly scooped inward and your buttocks squeezed.

AVOID

- Allowing your back to do the work by extending out of your hips.
- Lifting your hips so high that your weight shifts onto your neck.

1 Lie in supine position on the floor, your arms by your sides and lengthened toward your feet. Your legs should be bent, with your feet flat on the mat. Inhale to prepare.

2 Exhale, lifting your hips and spine off the floor, creating one long line from your knees to your shoulders. Keep your weight shifted over your feet.

3 Inhale, bringing your right knee toward your chest, your toe pointed.

4 Exhale, keeping your toe pointed, and lower your leg until your toe touches the mat. Be sure to keep your pelvis level.

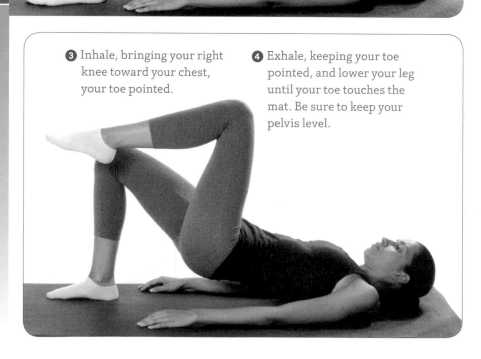

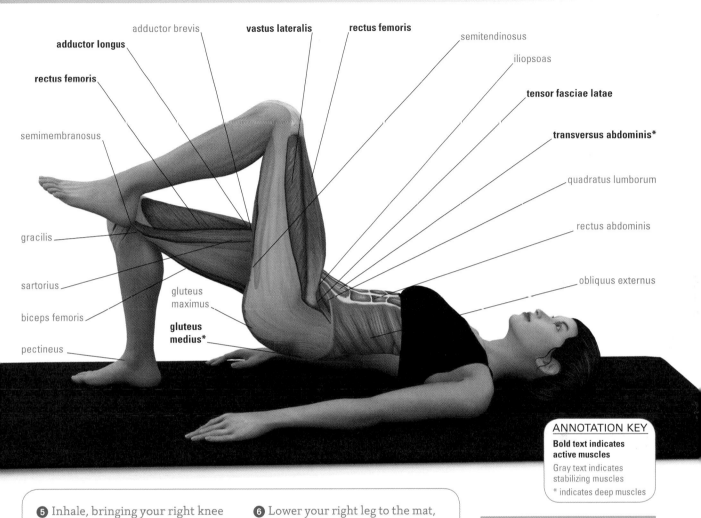

adductor brevis

vastus lateralis

rectus femoris

semitendinosus

adductor longus

iliopsoas

rectus femoris

tensor fasciae latae

semimembranosus

transversus abdominis*

quadratus lumborum

gracilis

rectus abdominis

sartorius

obliquus externus

biceps femoris

gluteus maximus

pectineus

gluteus medius*

ANNOTATION KEY

Bold text indicates active muscles

Gray text indicates stabilizing muscles

* indicates deep muscles

❺ Inhale, bringing your right knee toward the chest again. Repeat sequence four to five times.

❻ Lower your right leg to the mat, switch legs, and repeat the exercise with your left leg. Repeat sequence four to five times.

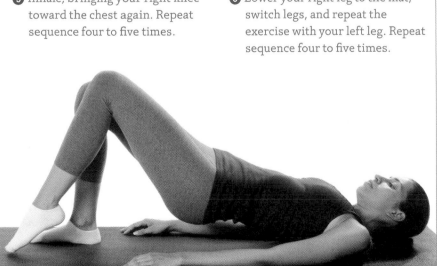

QUICK GUIDE

TARGET
• Hip extensor muscle

BENEFITS
• Increases stability in the pelvis and spine
• Increases hip flexor endurance

NOT ADVISABLE IF YOU HAVE
• Neck issues
• Severe knee injuries

NECK PULL

INTERMEDIATE

A more advanced version of the Roll-up exercise, the Neck Pull builds on principles that you've already mastered to target and strengthen the abdominal muscles. Rely on your torso to bring the body into a C curve, slowly rolling up and then back down the spine.

BEST FOR

- gluteus medius
- gluteus maximus
- rectus abdominis
- transversus abdominis
- quadratus lumborum
- semitendinosus
- semimembranosus
- biceps femoris
- iliopsoas
- rectus femoris
- sartorius
- tensor fasciae latae
- pectineus
- adductor longus
- adductor brevis
- gracilis

1 Lie in supine position on the floor with your hands behind your head and your elbows bent and to the side. Your legs should be straight and abducted slightly apart.

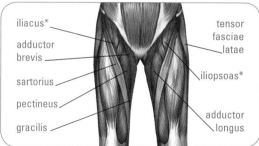

iliacus*
adductor brevis
sartorius
pectineus
gracilis
tensor fasciae latae
iliopsoas*
adductor longus

2 Inhale, lengthening the back of your neck and using your abdominals to curl your head and shoulders off the mat.

ANNOTATION KEY

Bold text indicates active muscles

Gray text indicates stabilizing muscles

*indicates deep muscles

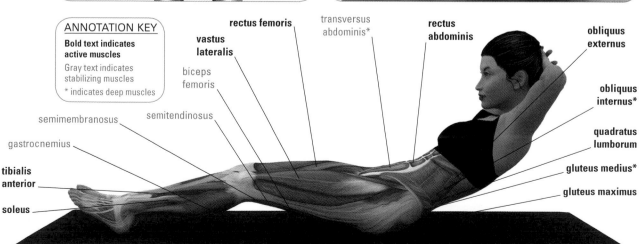

rectus femoris
vastus lateralis
biceps femoris
semitendinosus
semimembranosus
gastrocnemius
tibialis anterior
soleus
transversus abdominis*
rectus abdominis
obliquus externus
obliquus internus*
quadratus lumborum
gluteus medius*
gluteus maximus

DO IT RIGHT

LOOK FOR
- Focusing on your abdominals throughout the exercise while articulating through your spine.
- The Neck Pull is a more progressive version of the Roll-up, so take your time with the progression.
- Keeping your neck elongated and relaxed.

AVOID
- Pulling on your neck (despite the name of the exercise).

3 Exhale, drawing your navel into your spine and leading with your head. Articulate your upper body as you bring your torso off the mat and over your knees, creating a C curve in your back.

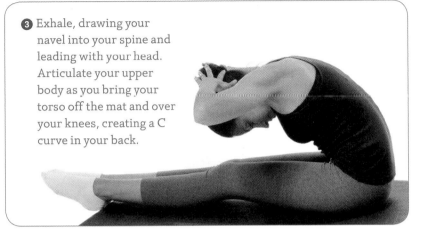

4 Inhale, stacking the spine into the neutral position, sitting up straight from your hips to your shoulders.

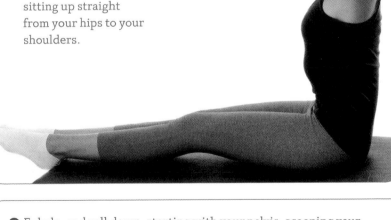

QUICK GUIDE

TARGET
- Abdominal muscles

BENEFITS
- Mobilizes the spine in flexion
- Strengthens the abdominals

NOT ADVISABLE IF YOU HAVE
- Cervical issues
- A herniated disk

5 Exhale, and roll down, starting with your pelvis, scooping your abdominals until you return to the starting position. Repeat sequence four to six times.

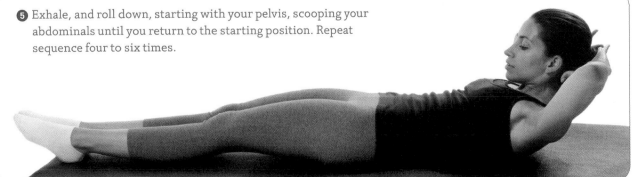

THE HUNDRED II

Another, more advanced version of a previous exercise, the intermediate Hundred is designed to build endurance and refine breathing technique. Ensure that your abdominals are properly engaged before starting the arm movement and repetition.

BEST FOR

- rectus abdominis
- gluteus maximus
- deltoideus
- biceps brachii
- triceps brachii
- extensor digitorum
- sternocleidomastoideus

❶ Lie in supine position on the floor with your arms outstretched beside your body. Your legs should be adducted together, your knees bent and raised in the tabletop position.

❷ Inhale, using your abdominals to lift your head, neck, and shoulders while lengthening your arms.

DO IT RIGHT

LOOK FOR
- Inhaling through the nose and exhaling through the mouth, focusing on your breathing throughout the exercise.

AVOID
- Leading with your head; keep your neck long and relaxed, allowing your abdominals to hold you up instead.

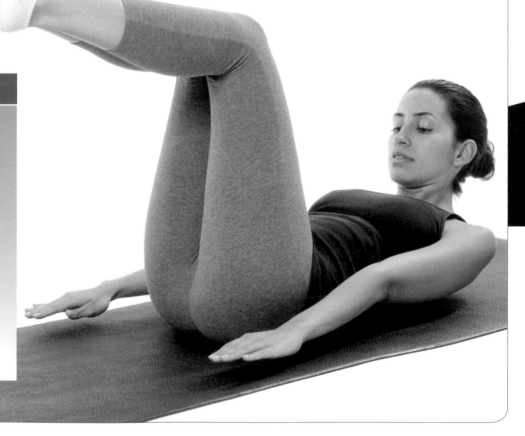

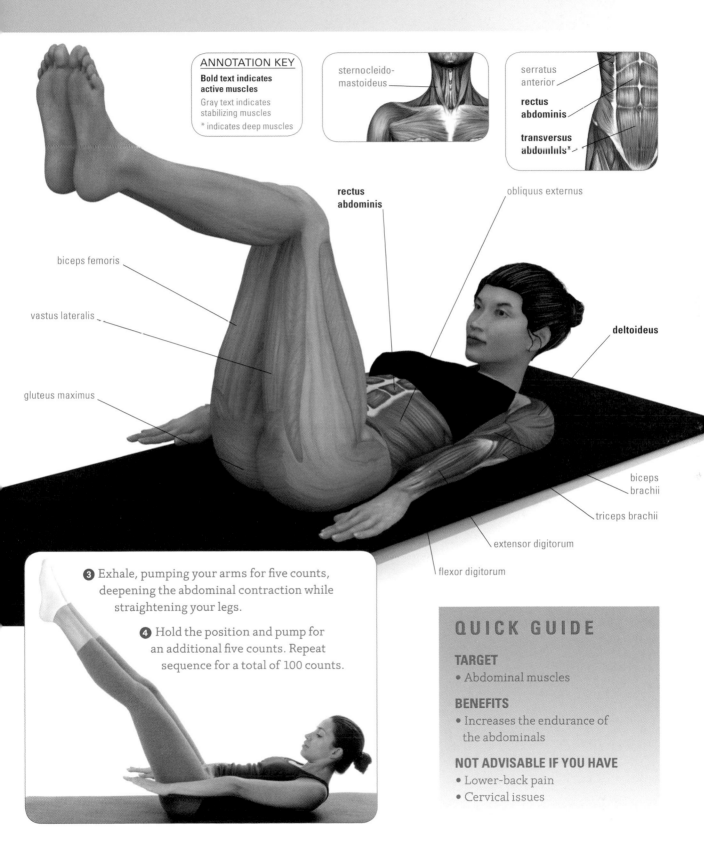

ANNOTATION KEY
Bold text indicates active muscles
Gray text indicates stabilizing muscles
* indicates deep muscles

sternocleido-mastoideus

serratus anterior
rectus abdominis
transversus abdominis

rectus abdominis

obliquus externus

biceps femoris

vastus lateralis

gluteus maximus

deltoideus

biceps brachii

triceps brachii

extensor digitorum

flexor digitorum

❸ Exhale, pumping your arms for five counts, deepening the abdominal contraction while straightening your legs.

❹ Hold the position and pump for an additional five counts. Repeat sequence for a total of 100 counts.

QUICK GUIDE

TARGET
• Abdominal muscles

BENEFITS
• Increases the endurance of the abdominals

NOT ADVISABLE IF YOU HAVE
• Lower-back pain
• Cervical issues

SAMPLE SEQUENCES

INTERMEDIATE

This group of exercises uses the base work that you developed from the Beginner section and incorporates more skilled techniques and movements. You should be able to perform these exercises with precision and control to avoid injury and provide yourself with the most benefit from your workout. Perform each exercise four to six times. Follow the breathing cues as you go through the movements; they are included to not only aid in the proper muscle recruitment but also to

BUILDING A BETTER CORE I

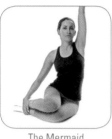
The Mermaid

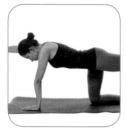
Plank with Leg Lift

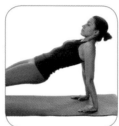
Leg Pull-back

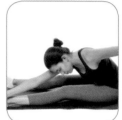
The Saw

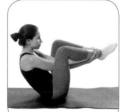
The Seal

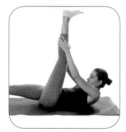
The Scissors

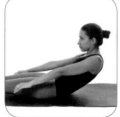
The Roll-up

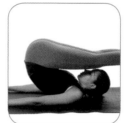
Rollover/Hip Up

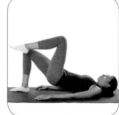
Bridge II

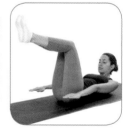
The Hundred II

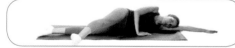
Side Kick II

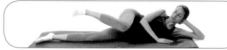
Bicycle Kick

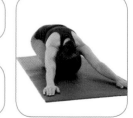
Child's Pose

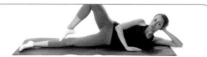
Side Passé

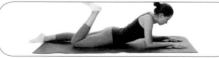
Single-leg Kick

STRETCHES

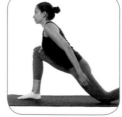
Hip Flexor Stretch

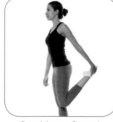
Quadriceps Stretch

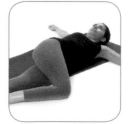
Spine Stretch I

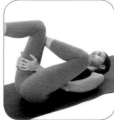
Piriformis Stretch

provide flow to your movements. Stretching after each workout is recommended for overall flexibility and muscle elongation. The Intermediate exercise series focuses on the flexion of the spine. The head is lifted in quite a few of these exercises, a move that relies on the engagement of the abdominal muscles. If you are experiencing neck pain while you perform these exercises, start with a folded towel under your head for additional support until you master lifting the torso with your abdominals—not your neck.

BUILDING A BETTER CORE II

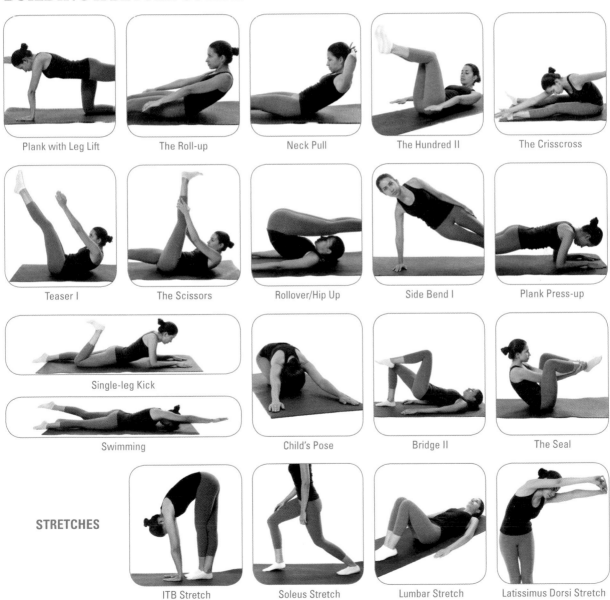

Plank with Leg Lift

The Roll-up

Neck Pull

The Hundred II

The Crisscross

Teaser I

The Scissors

Rollover/Hip Up

Side Bend I

Plank Press-up

Single-leg Kick

Swimming

Child's Pose

Bridge II

The Seal

STRETCHES

ITB Stretch

Soleus Stretch

Lumbar Stretch

Latissimus Dorsi Stretch

THE TWIST

ADVANCED

The Twist is a comprehensive way to work out the entire body while working on control and balance. The Twist gives special attention to the shoulder and abdominal muscles and also helps to whittle a defined waistline.

BEST FOR

- latissimus dorsi
- rectus abdominis
- obliquus internus
- obliquus externus
- transversus abdominis
- adductor magnus
- adductor longus
- deltoideus

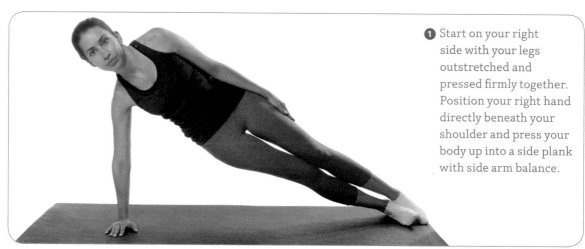

❶ Start on your right side with your legs outstretched and pressed firmly together. Position your right hand directly beneath your shoulder and press your body up into a side plank with side arm balance.

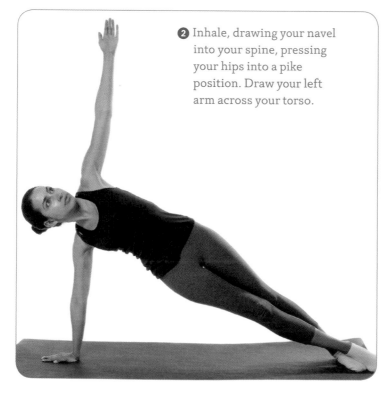

❷ Inhale, drawing your navel into your spine, pressing your hips into a pike position. Draw your left arm across your torso.

QUICK GUIDE

TARGET
- Shoulder
- Abdominal muscles

BENEFITS
- A total-body workout
- Builds endurance

NOT ADVISABLE IF YOU HAVE
- Shoulder issues
- Back pain
- Wrist injury

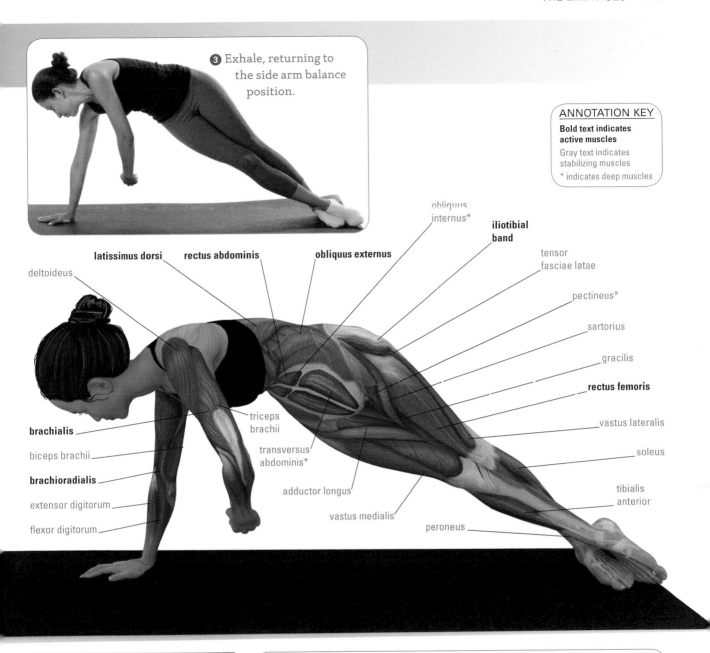

❸ Exhale, returning to the side arm balance position.

obliquus internus*

iliotibial band

tensor fasciae latae

pectineus*

sartorius

gracilis

rectus femoris

vastus lateralis

soleus

tibialis anterior

peroneus

vastus medialis

adductor longus

transversus abdominis*

triceps brachii

obliquus externus

rectus abdominis

latissimus dorsi

deltoideus

brachialis

biceps brachii

brachioradialis

extensor digitorum

flexor digitorum

DO IT RIGHT

LOOK FOR
- Elongating limbs as much as possible.
- Maintaining shoulder stability.
- Lifting your hips up high to reduce the amount of weight on your upper body.

AVOID
- Allowing your shoulder to sink into its socket.

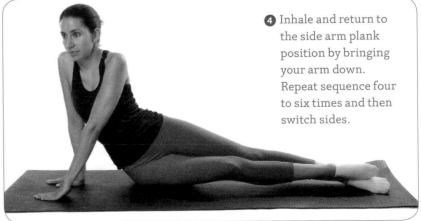

❹ Inhale and return to the side arm plank position by bringing your arm down. Repeat sequence four to six times and then switch sides.

SIDE KICK II

ADVANCED

Great for toning the lower body, the Side Kick II is also the perfect way to focus on the spine and build its stability. These movements exemplify the principle of articulation—challenge yourself to make each kick a smooth and separate movement.

DO IT RIGHT

LOOK FOR
- Pressing your weight into the floor with your elbow.
- Keeping your neck elongated and relaxed.

AVOID
- Allowing your hips and body to move back and forth while legs are in motion.

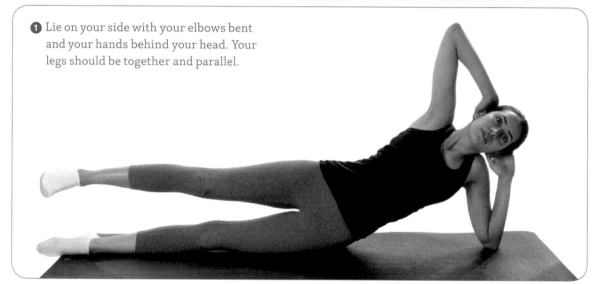

1 Lie on your side with your elbows bent and your hands behind your head. Your legs should be together and parallel.

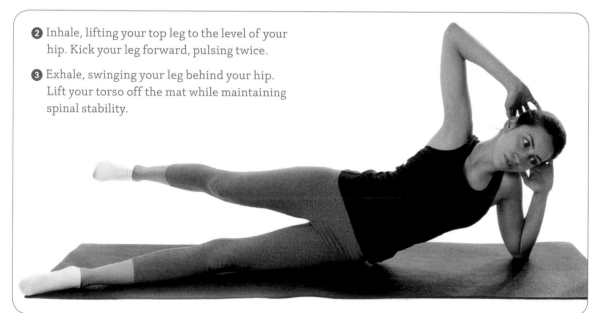

2 Inhale, lifting your top leg to the level of your hip. Kick your leg forward, pulsing twice.

3 Exhale, swinging your leg behind your hip. Lift your torso off the mat while maintaining spinal stability.

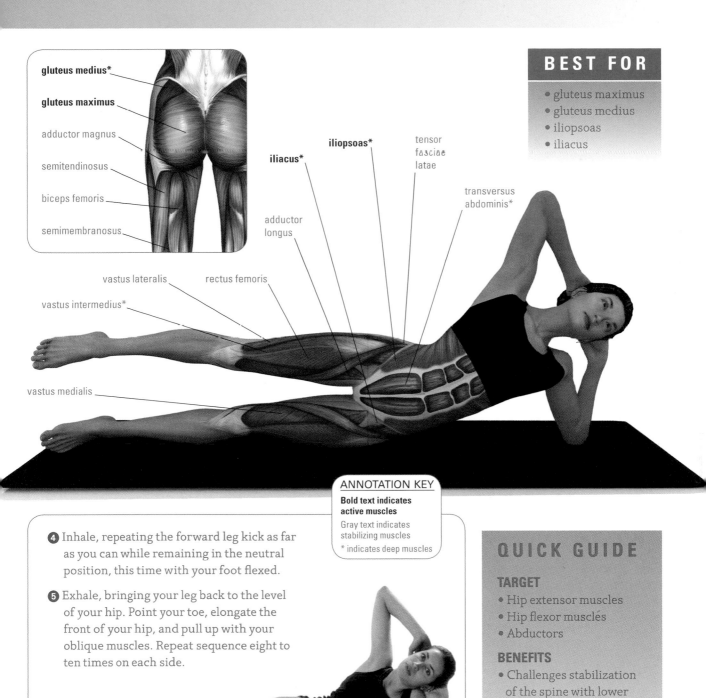

gluteus medius*

gluteus maximus

adductor magnus

semitendinosus

biceps femoris

semimembranosus

vastus lateralis

vastus intermedius*

vastus medialis

iliacus*

adductor longus

iliopsoas*

rectus femoris

tensor fasciae latae

transversus abdominis*

ANNOTATION KEY

Bold text indicates active muscles

Gray text indicates stabilizing muscles

* indicates deep muscles

④ Inhale, repeating the forward leg kick as far as you can while remaining in the neutral position, this time with your foot flexed.

⑤ Exhale, bringing your leg back to the level of your hip. Point your toe, elongate the front of your hip, and pull up with your oblique muscles. Repeat sequence eight to ten times on each side.

QUICK GUIDE

TARGET

- Hip extensor muscles
- Hip flexor muscles
- Abductors

BENEFITS

- Challenges stabilization of the spine with lower extremity movement

NOT ADVISABLE IF YOU HAVE

- Shoulder issues. If this is the case, keep your head flat during the exercise.

TEASER II

ADVANCED

This demanding but effective exercise requires absolute control over the abdominal muscles. The Teaser II benefits the spine as well because the rolling movement encourages flexibility and elongation.

BEST FOR

- iliopsoas
- iliacus
- rectus abdominis
- obliquus externus
- obliquus internus
- transversus abdominis

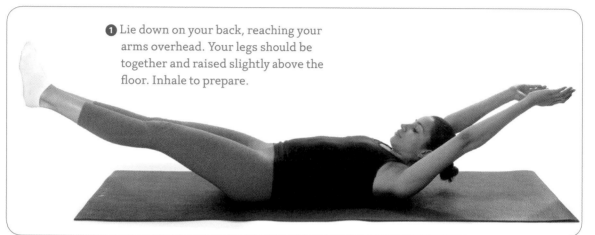

❶ Lie down on your back, reaching your arms overhead. Your legs should be together and raised slightly above the floor. Inhale to prepare.

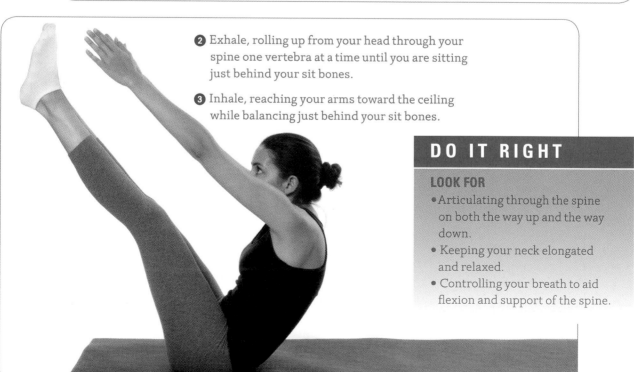

❷ Exhale, rolling up from your head through your spine one vertebra at a time until you are sitting just behind your sit bones.

❸ Inhale, reaching your arms toward the ceiling while balancing just behind your sit bones.

DO IT RIGHT

LOOK FOR
- Articulating through the spine on both the way up and the way down.
- Keeping your neck elongated and relaxed.
- Controlling your breath to aid flexion and support of the spine.

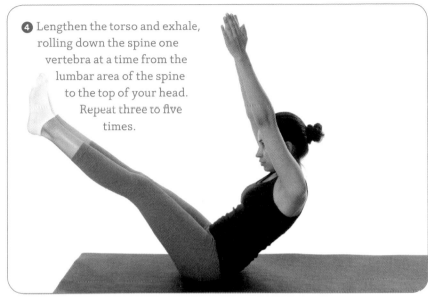

4 Lengthen the torso and exhale, rolling down the spine one vertebra at a time from the lumbar area of the spine to the top of your head. Repeat three to five times.

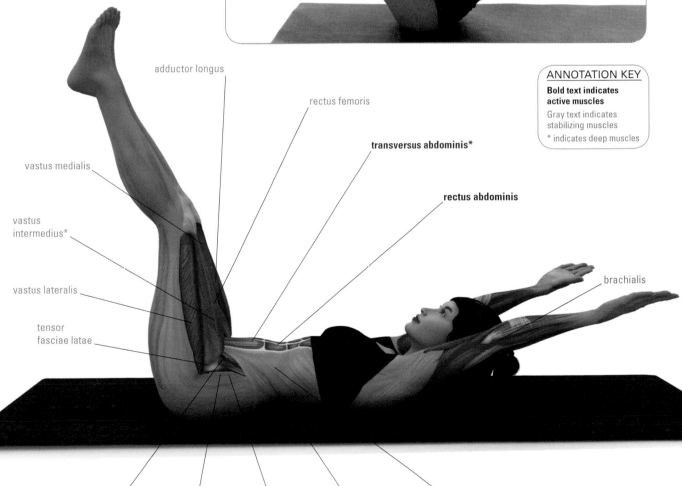

adductor longus

rectus femoris

transversus abdominis*

rectus abdominis

vastus medialis

vastus intermedius*

brachialis

vastus lateralis

tensor fasciae latae

pectineus*   **iliacus***   **iliopsoas***   **obliquus internus***   **obliquus externus**

OPEN-LEG ROCKER

ADVANCED

With a focus on the abdominal and hip muscles, the Open-leg Rocker may seem deceptively simple. But this exercise produces major results. By controlling the distribution of your weight as you roll back on your spine, you will successfully strengthen the targeted muscles and increase flexibility.

BEST FOR

- rectus abdominis
- obliquus internus
- obliquus externus
- transversus abdominis
- iliopsoas
- iliacus

1 Sitting on the mat, hold your legs or calves. Your legs should be abducted and parallel, with your knees straight.

2 Inhale, scooping your abdominals in while rolling off your sit bones. Do not allow your weight to extend beyond mid scapula.

3 Exhale, rolling your body back to the starting position. Repeat six to eight times.

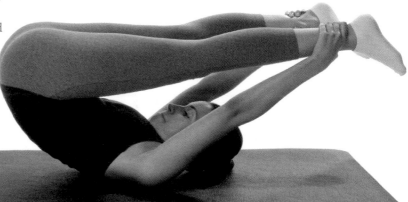

DO IT RIGHT

LOOK FOR
- Deeply scooped abdominal muscles.
- Keeping your neck elongated and relaxed.

AVOID
- Rolling back onto your neck. If you have trouble stopping, bend your knees slightly as you return to the starting position.

QUICK GUIDE

TARGET
- Abdominal muscles
- Hip flexors

BENEFITS
- Develops stability in the spine through the rocking motion

NOT ADVISABLE IF YOU HAVE
- A herniated disk

rectus abdominis

transversus abdominis*

obliquus internus*

obliquus externus

iliacus*

iliopsoas*

ANNOTATION KEY

Bold text indicates active muscles

Gray text indicates stabilizing muscles

* indicates deep muscles

DOUBLE-LEG KICK

ADVANCED

This Double-leg Kick, which is performed in the prone position, encourages both the chest and the back to open in order to maintain maximum stability. The added stability frees you to concentrate on working the muscles of the thighs and buttocks.

DO IT RIGHT

LOOK FOR
- Drawing your abdominals in toward your spine throughout the entire exercise.
- Keeping your neck elongated and relaxed.

AVOID
- Moving too quickly.
- Lifting hips off mat.

❶ Lying prone on the floor with your legs adducted and parallel, flex your knees. Bend your arms and place your hands, interlaced, in the small of your back. Allow your elbows to drop down to the mat.

❷ Exhale, pulsing your knees for three breaths while keeping your pelvis stable.

❸ Inhale, and stretch your spine and hips, separating your legs and reaching your arms back toward your hips. Look forward through the stretch. Extend your arms far behind your back, squeezing your shoulder blades together to open up your chest.

QUICK GUIDE

TARGET
- Erector spinae
- Hip extensors

BENEFITS
- Opens your chest, strengthens your back, and tones thighs and buttocks

NOT ADVISABLE IF YOU HAVE
- Cervical issues
- Sharp lower-back pain

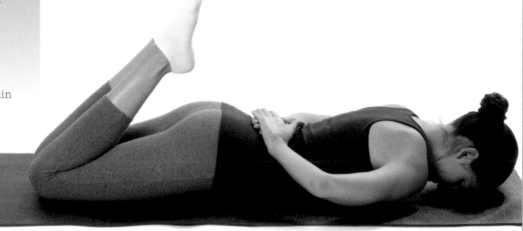

4 Exhale, bringing your legs together and bending your knees to return to your starting position. Bend your elbows and bring your hands to the small of your back.

5 Repeat sequence five to six times.

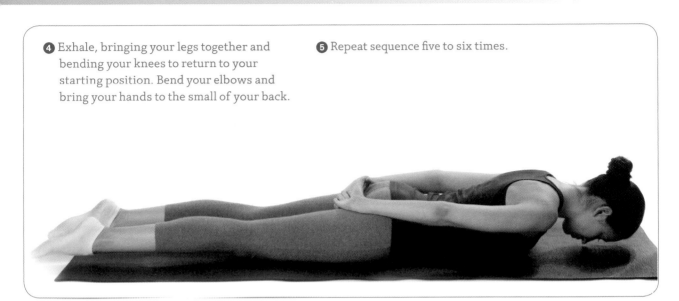

BEST FOR

- latissimus dorsi
- erector spinae
- gluteus maximus
- trapezius

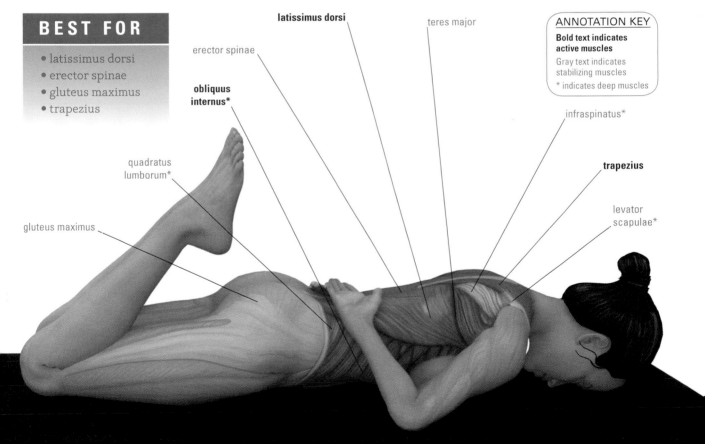

latissimus dorsi

teres major

erector spinae

ANNOTATION KEY
Bold text indicates active muscles
Gray text indicates stabilizing muscles
* indicates deep muscles

obliquus internus*

infraspinatus*

quadratus lumborum*

trapezius

gluteus maximus

levator scapulae*

SHORT PLANK

ADVANCED

The Short Plank effectively targets the upper body. Similar to a traditional push-up, the aim of this exercise is the constant lengthening of the spine and precise, deliberate breathing.

BEST FOR

- pectoralis major
- serratus anterior
- rectus abdominis
- obliquus internus
- obliquus externus
- transversus abdominis
- gluteus maximus
- deltoideus
- latissimus dorsi
- trapezius

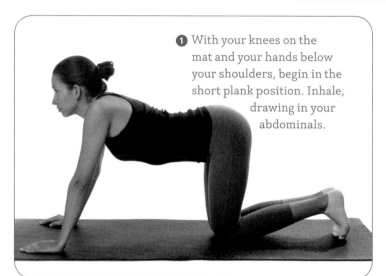

1 With your knees on the mat and your hands below your shoulders, begin in the short plank position. Inhale, drawing in your abdominals.

QUICK GUIDE

TARGET
- Pectoralis major
- Abdominal muscles
- Hip extensor muscles

BENEFITS
- Strengthens shoulder stabilizers with isometric exercise

NOT ADVISABLE IF YOU HAVE
- Unstable shoulders
- Wrist injury

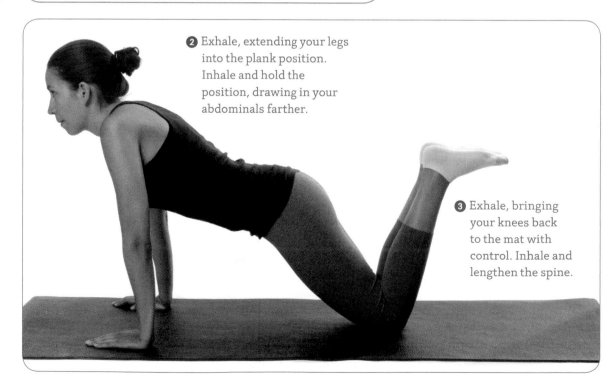

2 Exhale, extending your legs into the plank position. Inhale and hold the position, drawing in your abdominals farther.

3 Exhale, bringing your knees back to the mat with control. Inhale and lengthen the spine.

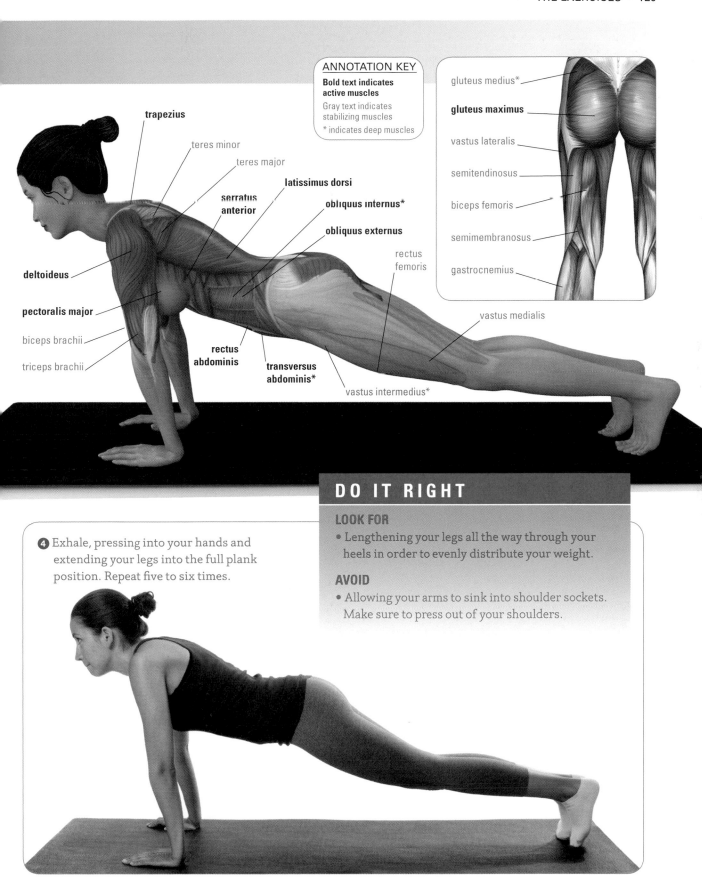

ANNOTATION KEY
Bold text indicates active muscles
Gray text indicates stabilizing muscles
* indicates deep muscles

trapezius

teres minor

teres major

latissimus dorsi

serratus anterior

obliquus internus*

obliquus externus

rectus femoris

deltoideus

pectoralis major

biceps brachii

triceps brachii

rectus abdominis

transversus abdominis*

vastus intermedius*

gluteus medius*

gluteus maximus

vastus lateralis

semitendinosus

biceps femoris

semimembranosus

gastrocnemius

vastus medialis

❹ Exhale, pressing into your hands and extending your legs into the full plank position. Repeat five to six times.

DO IT RIGHT

LOOK FOR
• Lengthening your legs all the way through your heels in order to evenly distribute your weight.

AVOID
• Allowing your arms to sink into shoulder sockets. Make sure to press out of your shoulders.

LEG PULL-DOWN

ADVANCED

The Leg Pull-down requires a high level of balance and control over the arms and legs. During the leg extensions, your spine should remain long and straight and seem to "float" over your body.

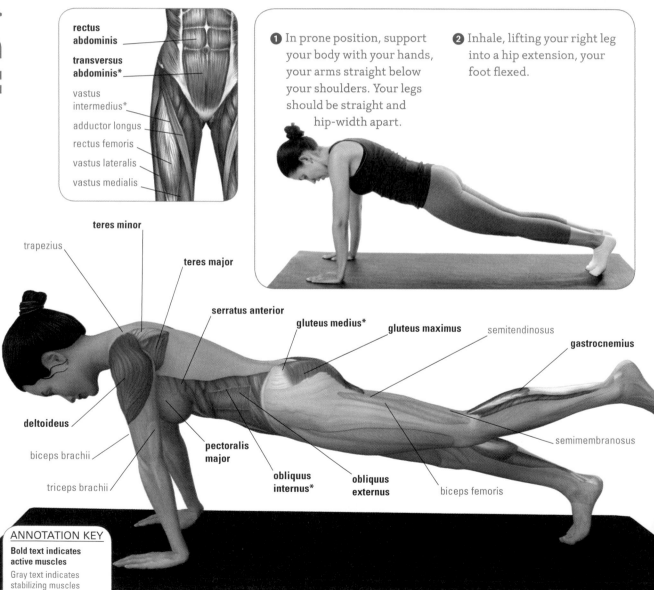

DO IT RIGHT

LOOK FOR
- Keeping your hips in line with your shoulders and ankles to achieve optimal weight distribution.
- Keeping your neck elongated and relaxed.

AVOID
- Sagging your lower back as you fatigue.

rectus abdominis

transversus abdominis*

vastus intermedius*

adductor longus

rectus femoris

vastus lateralis

vastus medialis

❶ In prone position, support your body with your hands, your arms straight below your shoulders. Your legs should be straight and hip-width apart.

❷ Inhale, lifting your right leg into a hip extension, your foot flexed.

teres minor

trapezius

teres major

serratus anterior

gluteus medius*

gluteus maximus

semitendinosus

gastrocnemius

deltoideus

biceps brachii

pectoralis major

triceps brachii

obliquus internus*

obliquus externus

biceps femoris

semimembranosus

ANNOTATION KEY
Bold text indicates active muscles
Gray text indicates stabilizing muscles
* indicates deep muscles

3 Exhale, pointing your right foot and lengthening your body as your weight transfers from your arms to your left foot, stretching through your heel.

BEST FOR

- pectoralis major
- serratus anterior
- deltoideus
- rectus abdominis
- obliquus internus
- obliquus externus
- transversus abdominis
- gluteus maximus
- gastrocnemius

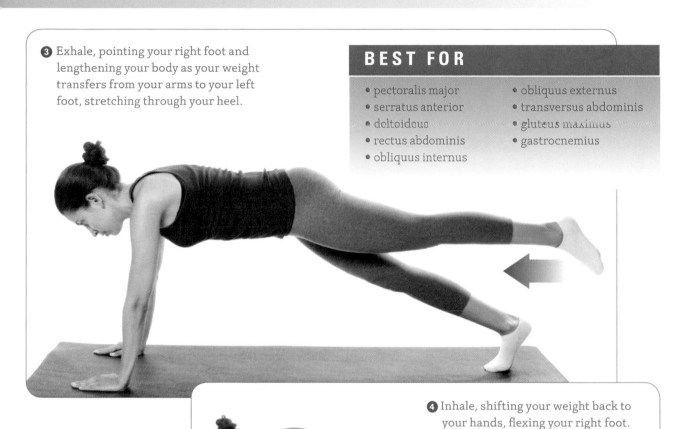

4 Inhale, shifting your weight back to your hands, flexing your right foot.

5 Exhale, bringing your right leg back to the starting position. Switch legs and repeat five to six times on each side.

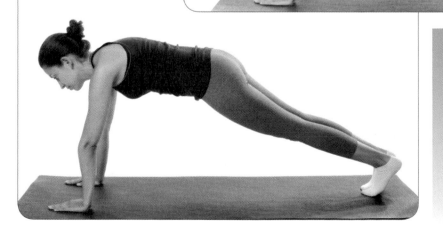

QUICK GUIDE

TARGET
- Abdominal muscles
- Shoulder girdle stabilizers

BENEFITS
- Stabilizes the spine against gravity

NOT ADVISABLE IF YOU HAVE
- Shoulder issues

HIP TWIST

ADVANCED

Another excellent, intense workout for the lower body, the Hip Twist demands control of the legs and directly targets the abdominal muscles.

BEST FOR

- tensor fasciae latae
- rectus femoris
- vastus lateralis
- sartorius
- biceps femoris
- gluteus maximus
- gluteus medius
- iliotibial band
- vastus medialis
- vastus intermedius
- adductor longus

❶ Begin by sitting on the mat with your arms behind your body, supporting your weight. Legs should be parallel and raised to a high diagonal.

❷ Inhale, engaging your abdominals and shoulders for stabilization.

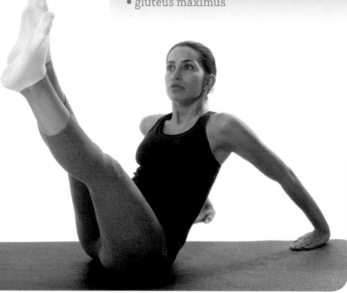

❺ Inhale, returning your legs to the starting position. Repeat four to six times.

❸ Exhale, and start to bring the legs across the body to one side.

❹ Exhale, continuing to circle the legs across the body and down as low as pelvic stabilization can be maintained.

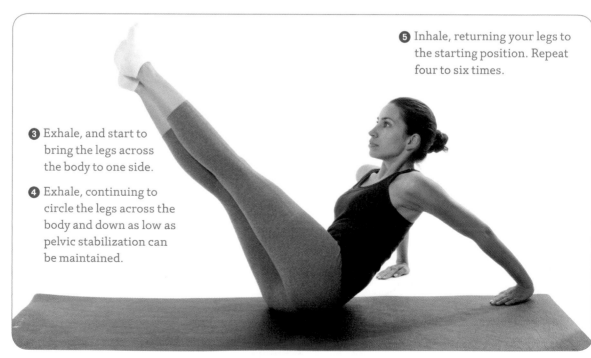

QUICK GUIDE

TARGET
• Abdominal muscles

BENEFITS
• Strengthens all four abdominals against gravity and weight of legs

NOT ADVISABLE IF YOU HAVE
• Back pain
• Hip instability

DO IT RIGHT

LOOK FOR
• Lengthening through your legs as you move from side to side.
• Pressing up out of your shoulders to better engage your torso.
• Elongating your neck.

AVOID
• Tensing your neck and shoulder muscles.

rectus abdominis

transversus abdominis*

vastus intermedius*

adductor longus

rectus femoris

vastus lateralis

obliquus externus

obliquus internus*

biceps femoris

iliotibial band

gluteus maximus

deltoideus

triceps brachii

biceps brachii

gluteus medius*

tensor fasciae latae

ANNOTATION KEY
Bold text indicates active muscles
Gray text indicates stabilizing muscles
* indicates deep muscles

SEAL WITH FOOT CLAP

ADVANCED

The Seal with Foot Clap helps you focus on achieving a high level of balance. Instead of targeting the body's superficial muscles, the advanced version of the Seal uses the pelvis and deep abdominal muscles to create and limit momentum as you roll on your spine.

DO IT RIGHT

LOOK FOR
• Allowing your momentum to help you roll backward.

AVOID
• Allowing your back to make a "thumping" sound—this indicates that you need to draw in the abdominals to make a smoother movement.
• Rolling too far back on your neck—stay on your shoulder blades.

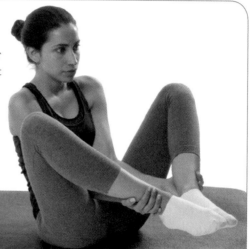

❶ Start by sitting up on your balance point position, balancing slightly behind your tailbone, with your knees bent and open to the sides.

❷ With your feet together and off the floor, grab your ankles from the insides of the legs. Clap your feet together three times.

QUICK GUIDE

TARGET
• Pelvic stabilizer muscles
• Deep abdominal muscles

NOT ADVISABLE IF YOU HAVE
• Intense neck pain
• Elbow pain

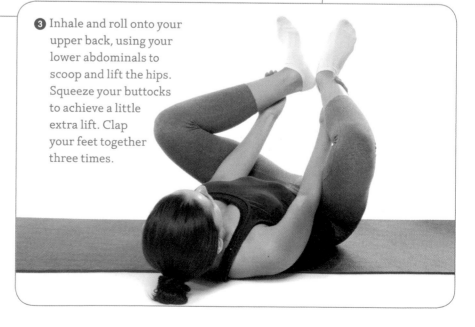

❸ Inhale and roll onto your upper back, using your lower abdominals to scoop and lift the hips. Squeeze your buttocks to achieve a little extra lift. Clap your feet together three times.

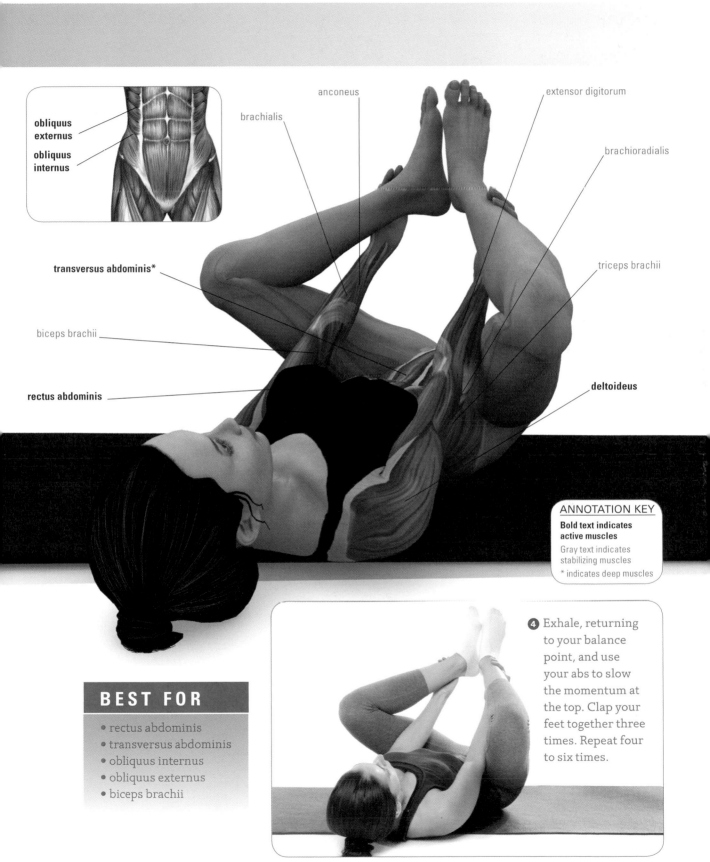

obliquus
externus

obliquus
internus

anconeus

brachialis

extensor digitorum

brachioradialis

transversus abdominis*

triceps brachii

biceps brachii

rectus abdominis

deltoideus

❹ Exhale, returning
to your balance
point, and use
your abs to slow
the momentum at
the top. Clap your
feet together three
times. Repeat four
to six times.

BEST FOR

• rectus abdominis
• transversus abdominis
• obliquus internus
• obliquus externus
• biceps brachii

SIDE BEND II

ADVANCED

The Side Bend II is a more specialized version of the Side Bend, and it addresses both the upper body and the abdominal muscles. You should attempt a long, smooth reach to achieve maximum stretch, as well as even weight distribution.

BEST FOR

- rectus abdominis
- obliquus externus
- rectus femoris
- tensor fasciae latae
- vastus lateralis
- adductor magnus
- adductor longus
- biceps femoris
- gluteus maximus

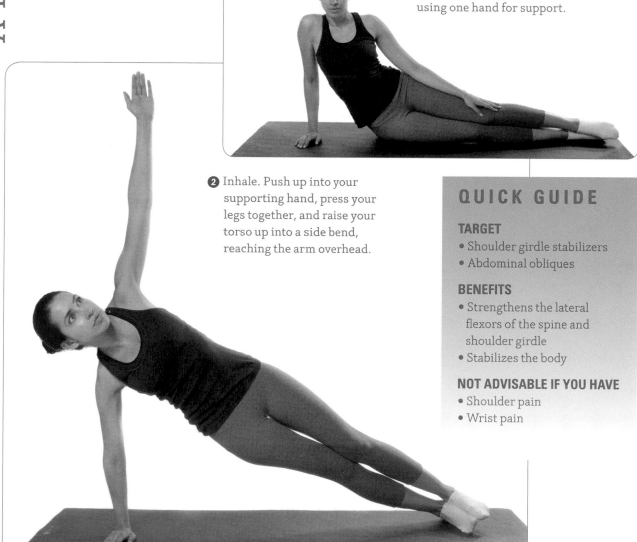

1 Begin in a half-lying position, your legs together and parallel to the mat, using one hand for support.

2 Inhale. Push up into your supporting hand, press your legs together, and raise your torso up into a side bend, reaching the arm overhead.

QUICK GUIDE

TARGET
- Shoulder girdle stabilizers
- Abdominal obliques

BENEFITS
- Strengthens the lateral flexors of the spine and shoulder girdle
- Stabilizes the body

NOT ADVISABLE IF YOU HAVE
- Shoulder pain
- Wrist pain

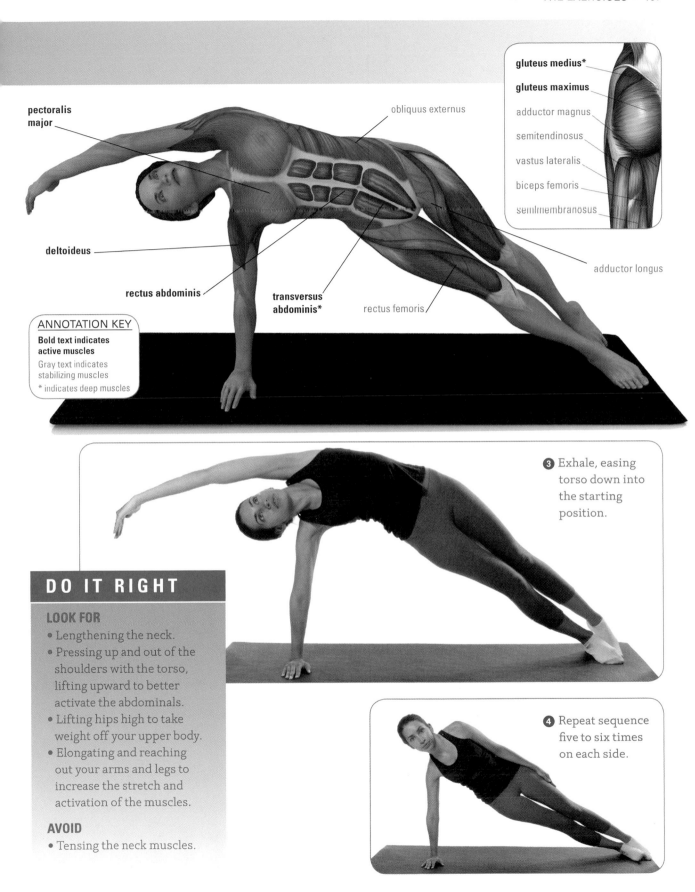

pectoralis major

obliquus externus

gluteus medius*

gluteus maximus

adductor magnus

semitendinosus

vastus lateralis

biceps femoris

semimembranosus

adductor longus

deltoideus

rectus abdominis

transversus abdominis*

rectus femoris

ANNOTATION KEY
Bold text indicates active muscles
Gray text indicates stabilizing muscles
* indicates deep muscles

❸ Exhale, easing torso down into the starting position.

DO IT RIGHT

LOOK FOR
- Lengthening the neck.
- Pressing up and out of the shoulders with the torso, lifting upward to better activate the abdominals.
- Lifting hips high to take weight off your upper body.
- Elongating and reaching out your arms and legs to increase the stretch and activation of the muscles.

AVOID
- Tensing the neck muscles.

❹ Repeat sequence five to six times on each side.

PUSH-UP

ADVANCED

The classic Push-up is an enduring cornerstone of any fitness plan. By rolling up and down your spine at the beginning and end, you encourage length and space in the spine and prepare your entire body for precise, controlled movement.

BEST FOR

- rectus abdominis
- transversus abdominis
- obliquus externus
- obliquus internus
- triceps brachii
- trapezius
- gluteus maximus
- pectoralis major

❶ Standing at the back of your mat, inhale and pull your navel to your spine.

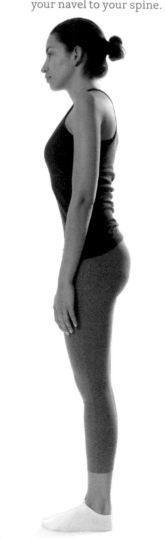

❷ Exhale as you roll down one vertebra at a time and walk your hands out until they are directly beneath the shoulders in the plank position.

❸ Inhale and set your body by drawing your abdominals to your spine. Squeeze your buttocks and legs together and stretch out of your heels, bringing your body into a straight line.

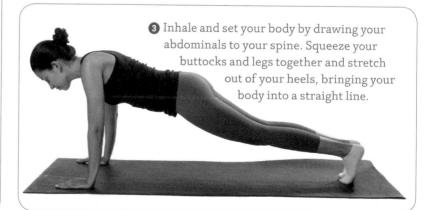

DO IT RIGHT

LOOK FOR
- Keeping your head and neck long and relaxed as you perform the Push-up.
- Squeezing the buttocks muscles and drawing in the abdominals for stability.

AVOID
- Letting your shoulders hunch up toward your ears.

QUICK GUIDE

TARGET
- Pectoralis major
- Biceps
- Triceps

BENEFITS
- Strengthens the core stabilizers, shoulders, back, buttocks, and muscles of the chest

NOT ADVISABLE IF YOU HAVE
- Shoulder issues
- Wrist pain
- Lower-back pain

④ Exhale and inhale as you bend the elbows and lower your body downward and push upward. Repeat eight times.

⑤ Inhale as you lift your hips into the air and walk your hands back toward your feet. Exhale slowly, rolling up one vertebra at a time into your starting position. Repeat the entire exercise three times.

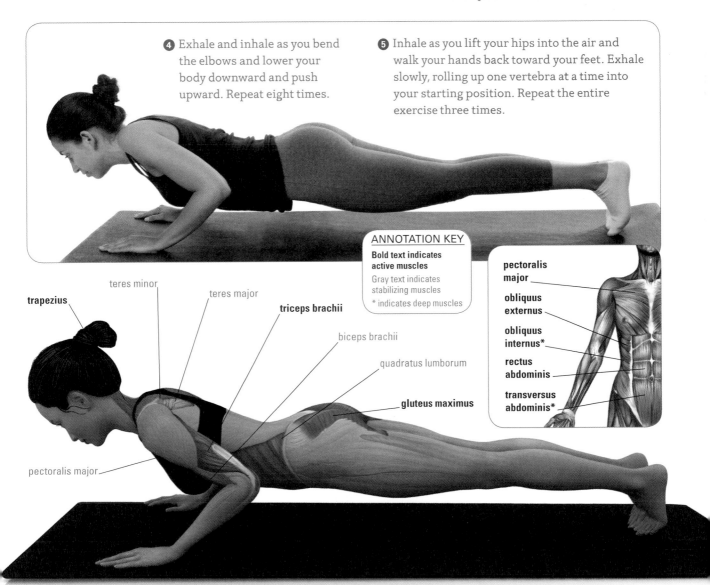

ANNOTATION KEY
Bold text indicates active muscles
Gray text indicates stabilizing muscles
* indicates deep muscles

trapezius
teres minor
teres major
triceps brachii
biceps brachii
quadratus lumborum
gluteus maximus
pectoralis major

pectoralis major
obliquus externus
obliquus internus*
rectus abdominis
transversus abdominis*

SIDE LEG LIFT

ADVANCED

The Side Leg Lift engages the oblique abdominal muscles and promotes lengthening of all of the major muscles. Take advantage of the opportunity to focus on body balance and stability.

DO IT RIGHT

LOOK FOR
- Squeezing buttocks before lifting to better stabilize the pelvis.
- Elongating neck and head to reduce stress and strain on the neck.
- Sliding the hand on the leg down far from the ears to elongate.

BEST FOR
- rectus abdominis
- transversus abdominis
- obliquus externus
- obliquus internus

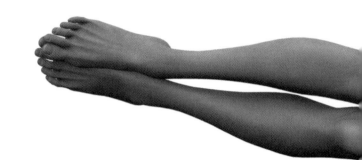

❶ Begin by lying on your side, one arm bent, supporting your head, the other flat along your thigh. Your legs are together and outstretched.

❷ Inhale to prepare.

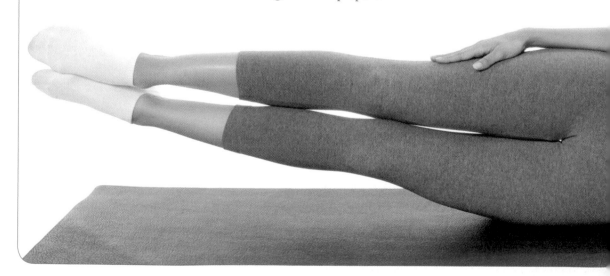

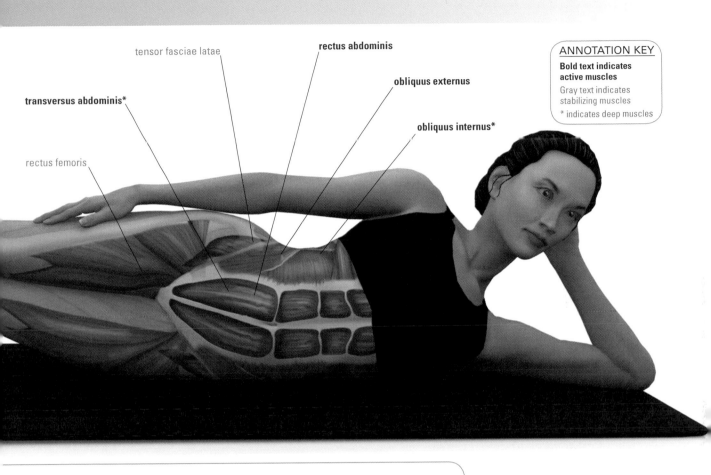

tensor fasciae latae

rectus abdominis

obliquus externus

transversus abdominis*

obliquus internus*

rectus femoris

3 Exhale, simultaneously lifting the head, shoulders, and legs.

4 Inhale, simultaneously lowering the legs and torso to the mat.

5 Repeat sequence four to six times on each side.

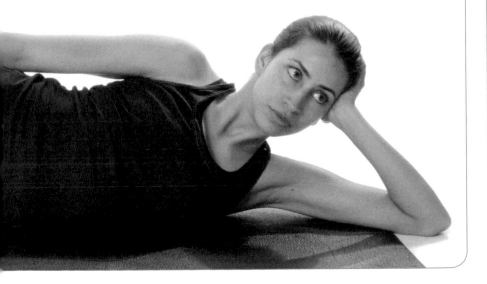

QUICK GUIDE

TARGET
• Oblique abdominals

BENEFITS
• Strengthens and stabilizes the body

NOT ADVISABLE IF YOU HAVE
• Lower-back pain

KNEELING SIDE KICK I

ADVANCED

The Kneeling Side Kick I, also called the Tall Kneeling Side Kick, stimulates several major muscle groups and encourages balance and muscle length throughout the entire body. Deep, full breathing as you proceed through these challenging movements will help you make the most of each stretch.

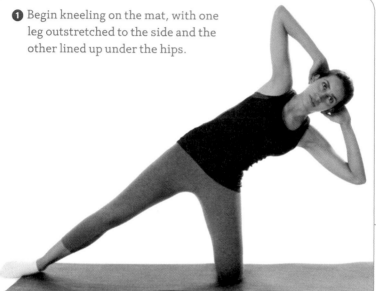

❶ Begin kneeling on the mat, with one leg outstretched to the side and the other lined up under the hips.

QUICK GUIDE

TARGET
- Abductor muscles
- Abdominal muscles
- Gluteal muscles

BENEFITS
- Trims the waistline

NOT ADVISABLE IF YOU HAVE
- Knee pain/injury
- Back pain

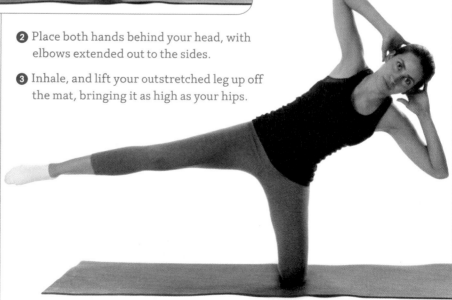

❷ Place both hands behind your head, with elbows extended out to the sides.

❸ Inhale, and lift your outstretched leg up off the mat, bringing it as high as your hips.

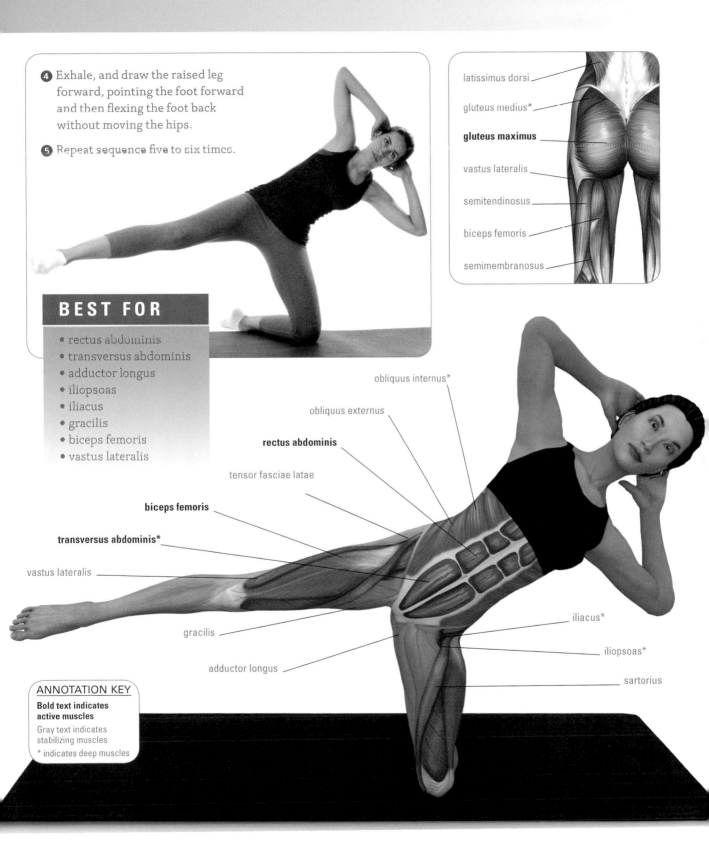

4 Exhale, and draw the raised leg forward, pointing the foot forward and then flexing the foot back without moving the hips.

5 Repeat sequence five to six times.

BEST FOR

- rectus abdominis
- transversus abdominis
- adductor longus
- iliopsoas
- iliacus
- gracilis
- biceps femoris
- vastus lateralis

latissimus dorsi
gluteus medius*
gluteus maximus
vastus lateralis
semitendinosus
biceps femoris
semimembranosus

obliquus internus*
obliquus externus
rectus abdominis
tensor fasciae latae
biceps femoris
transversus abdominis*
vastus lateralis
gracilis
adductor longus
iliacus*
iliopsoas*
sartorius

ANNOTATION KEY
Bold text indicates active muscles
Gray text indicates stabilizing muscles
* indicates deep muscles

OBLIQUE ROLL-DOWN

ADVANCED

❶ Begin by sitting on the mat with your arms extended, parallel to the floor, knees flexed and apart.

❷ Inhale, contracting your abdominals, drawing your navel to the spine, and lengthening the spine upward.

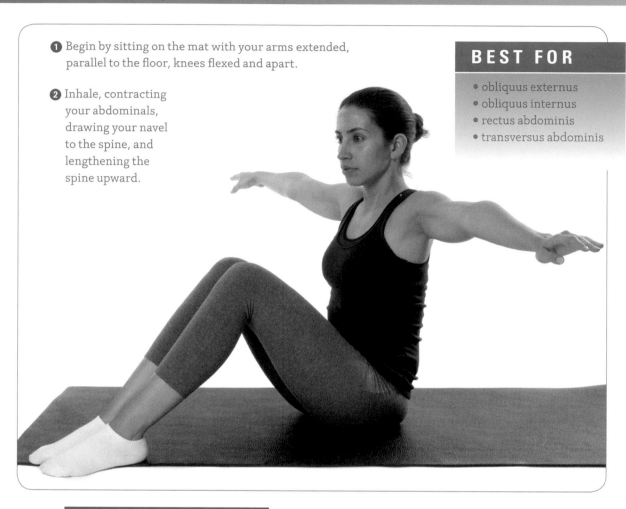

BEST FOR

- obliquus externus
- obliquus internus
- rectus abdominis
- transversus abdominis

DO IT RIGHT

LOOK FOR
- Lengthening the arms as you roll down to create opposition throughout the torso.
- Relaxing and lengthening the neck to prevent straining.
- Articulating through the spine while rolling up and down.
- Using a long, slow breath in and out to assist the movement.

AVOID
- Tensing your neck and shoulder muscles.

The C curve is paramount in the Oblique Roll-down. Monitor your abdominals and use your navel as a guide to ensure that those muscles are engaged and supporting the spine as you roll back and rotate.

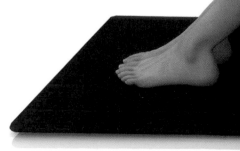

QUICK GUIDE

TARGET
• Oblique muscles

BENEFITS
• Targets the oblique abdominals while challenging the ability to maintain the C curve

NOT ADVISABLE IF YOU HAVE
• A herniated disk

③ Exhale, and roll backward while simultaneously rotating the torso to one side.

④ Inhale, maintaining spinal flexion, rotating your torso back to center.

⑤ Exhale, and rotate to the other side, deepening the abdominal contraction.

⑥ Inhale, return to center, and repeat sequence four to six times on each side.

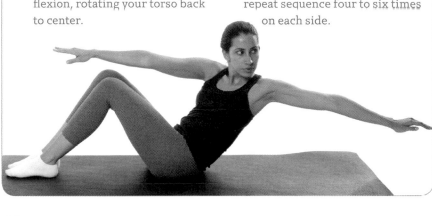

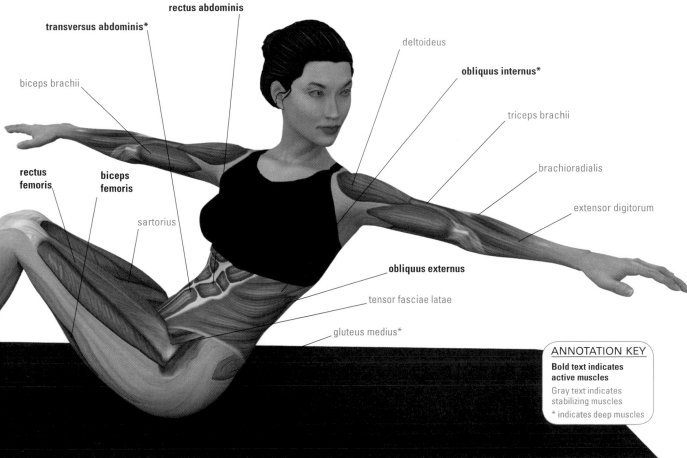

transversus abdominis*

rectus abdominis

biceps brachii

rectus femoris

biceps femoris

sartorius

deltoideus

obliquus internus*

triceps brachii

brachioradialis

extensor digitorum

obliquus externus

tensor fasciae latae

gluteus medius*

ANNOTATION KEY
Bold text indicates active muscles
Gray text indicates stabilizing muscles
* indicates deep muscles

BRIDGE III

ADVANCED

Building on the beginning and intermediate Bridge exercises, this third version of the exercise takes the Bridge movements to the limit, coordinating the legs, hips, and spine through successful use of the plank position.

BEST FOR

- gluteus maximus
- gluteus medialis
- quadriceps lumborum
- tensor fasciae latae
- rectus abdominis
- transversus abdominis
- semitendinosus
- semimembranosus
- biceps femoris

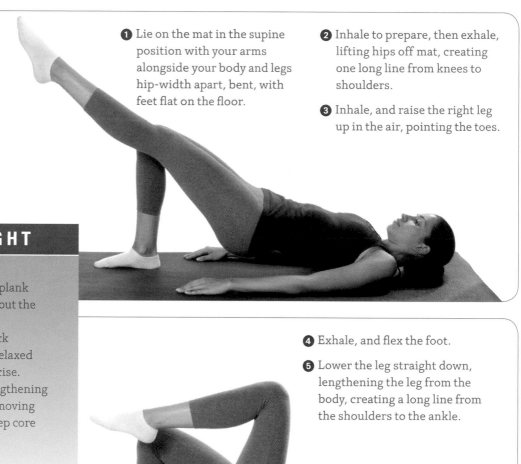

❶ Lie on the mat in the supine position with your arms alongside your body and legs hip-width apart, bent, with feet flat on the floor.

❷ Inhale to prepare, then exhale, lifting hips off mat, creating one long line from knees to shoulders.

❸ Inhale, and raise the right leg up in the air, pointing the toes.

❹ Exhale, and flex the foot.

❺ Lower the leg straight down, lengthening the leg from the body, creating a long line from the shoulders to the ankle.

DO IT RIGHT

LOOK FOR
- Maintaining the plank position throughout the motion.
- Keeping your neck lengthened and relaxed through the exercise.
- Reaching and lengthening of the leg that is moving to activate the deep core muscles.

AVOID
- Allowing the hips to lift or sink from plank position.

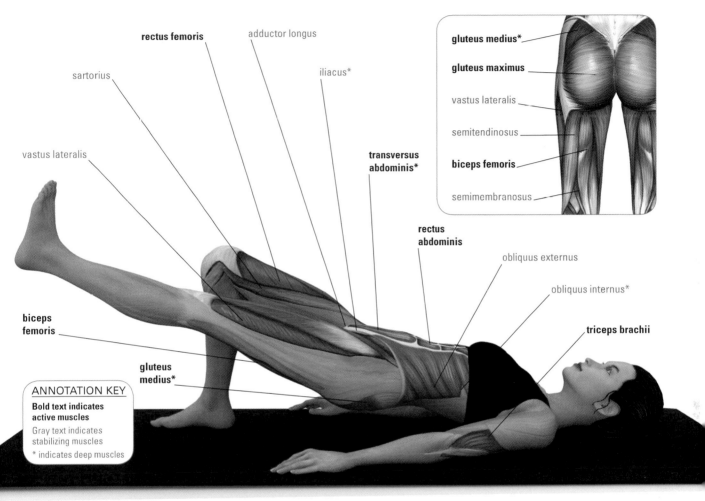

rectus femoris

adductor longus

iliacus*

sartorius

gluteus medius*

gluteus maximus

vastus lateralis

semitendinosus

biceps femoris

semimembranosus

vastus lateralis

transversus abdominis*

rectus abdominis

obliquus externus

obliquus internus*

biceps femoris

triceps brachii

gluteus medius*

ANNOTATION KEY
Bold text indicates active muscles
Gray text indicates stabilizing muscles
* indicates deep muscles

QUICK GUIDE

TARGET
• Hip extensors

BENEFITS
• Increases strength and endurance of hip flexors and stability of spine

NOT ADVISABLE IF YOU HAVE
• Neck issues

❻ Inhale, and draw the leg back up to the ceiling, pointing the toes.

❼ Repeat sequence four to six times, and then switch legs.

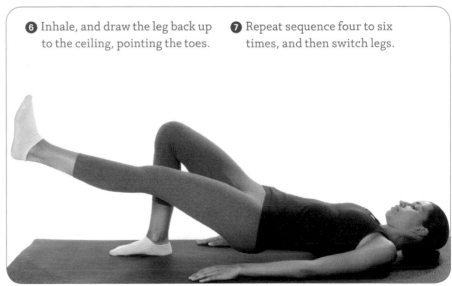

JACKKNIFE

ADVANCED

The Jackknife requires precise control over the abdominal, gluteal, and thigh muscles, which all benefit from this exercise. While the legs are extended into the air, the spine should be allowed to find as much length as possible.

BEST FOR

- rectus abdominis
- transversus abdominis
- gluteus maximus
- gluteus medius
- triceps brachii
- adductor longus

QUICK GUIDE

TARGET
- Abdominal muscles
- Inner thighs
- Buttocks

BENEFITS
- Strengthens hip and spine extensors
- Challenges stabilization of the spine against rotation

NOT ADVISABLE IF YOU HAVE
- Neck or shoulder issues
- A herniated disk

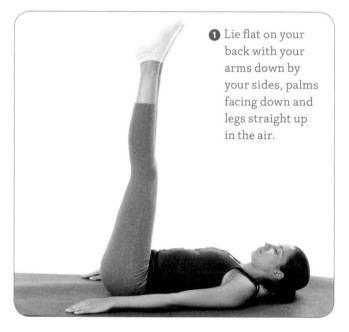

❶ Lie flat on your back with your arms down by your sides, palms facing down and legs straight up in the air.

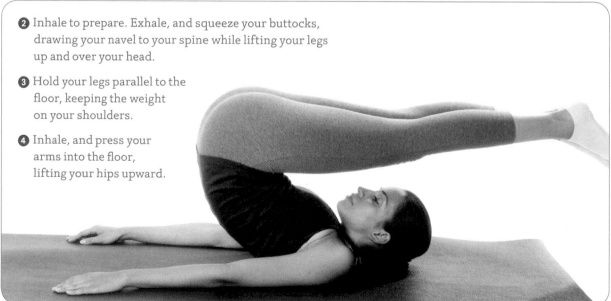

❷ Inhale to prepare. Exhale, and squeeze your buttocks, drawing your navel to your spine while lifting your legs up and over your head.

❸ Hold your legs parallel to the floor, keeping the weight on your shoulders.

❹ Inhale, and press your arms into the floor, lifting your hips upward.

⑤ Reach your legs straight into the air in a controlled, upward movement.

⑥ Exhale, rolling down your spine, and press your palms into the floor to slow movement.

⑦ Inhale, and lower your legs down toward the floor while keeping them straight.

⑧ Keeping your back flat on the floor, squeeze the inner thighs together.

⑨ Repeat sequence three to four times.

DO IT RIGHT

LOOK FOR
• Extending your limbs as long as possible in opposite directions.
• Squeezing your buttocks and drawing your navel into your spine throughout the exercise.
• Lengthening and relaxing your neck.

AVOID
• Raising your shoulders up to your ears.
• Rolling onto your neck. Your weight should rest on the back of your shoulders.
• Allowing the legs to separate.

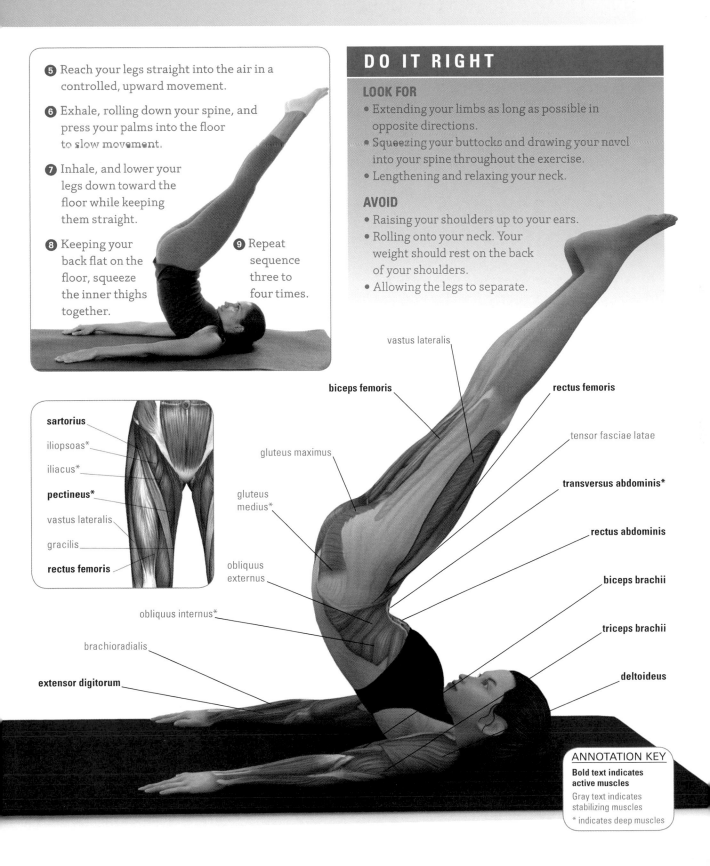

vastus lateralis

biceps femoris

gluteus maximus

gluteus medius*

obliquus externus

obliquus internus*

brachioradialis

extensor digitorum

sartorius
iliopsoas*
iliacus*
pectineus*
vastus lateralis
gracilis
rectus femoris

rectus femoris

tensor fasciae latae

transversus abdominis*

rectus abdominis

biceps brachii

triceps brachii

deltoideus

ANNOTATION KEY
Bold text indicates active muscles
Gray text indicates stabilizing muscles
* indicates deep muscles

CORKSCREW

ADVANCED

Complementary to the Jackknife, the Corkscrew engages the same muscles, but through different body positioning. Make sure that your circle motion is slow, precise, and no larger than necessary in order to maintain maximum stability.

BEST FOR

- pectineus
- adductor longus
- gracilis
- tensor fasciae latae
- sartorius
- rectus femoris
- iliacus
- iliopsoas
- vastus lateralis
- gluteus maximus
- rectus abdominis
- transversus abdominis
- obliquus externus
- obliquus internus

DO IT RIGHT

LOOK FOR

- Keeping the navel to your spine throughout the exercise.
- Making the circles as small as necessary to maintain stability.
- Relaxing and lengthening the neck.

AVOID

- Rolling back onto your neck.
- Allowing your back to arch off the mat.

❶ Lie down on the mat with your legs straight up in the air and arms down by your sides, your palms pressing into the floor.

❷ Inhale to prepare. Exhale, and pull your navel to your spine.

❸ Circle your legs to the left, down, around, and back to complete the circle.

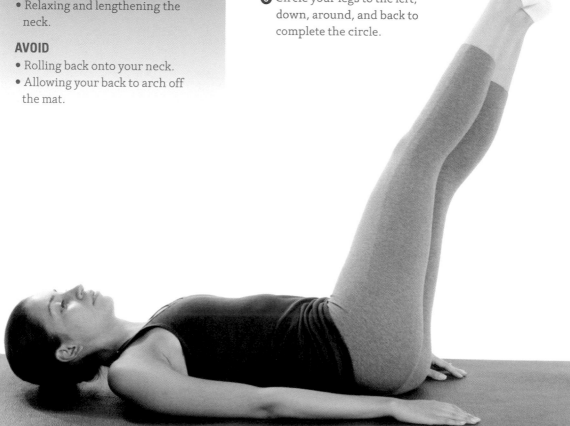

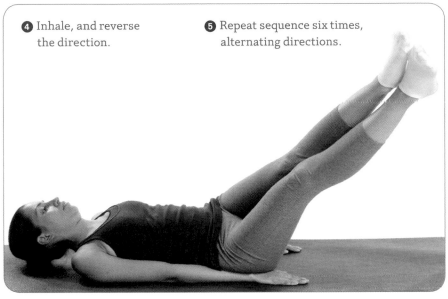

4 Inhale, and reverse the direction.

5 Repeat sequence six times, alternating directions.

QUICK GUIDE

TARGET
- Abdominal muscles
- Inner thighs
- Buttocks

BENEFITS
- Stretches the back muscles
- Improves balance

NOT ADVISABLE IF YOU HAVE
- Lower-back pain

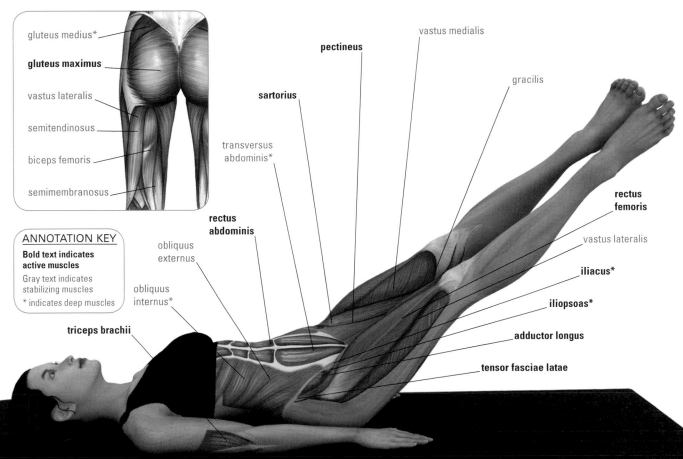

gluteus medius*

gluteus maximus

vastus lateralis

semitendinosus

biceps femoris

semimembranosus

vastus medialis

pectineus

gracilis

sartorius

transversus abdominis*

rectus femoris

vastus lateralis

iliacus*

iliopsoas*

adductor longus

tensor fasciae latae

rectus abdominis

obliquus externus

obliquus internus*

triceps brachii

ANNOTATION KEY
Bold text indicates active muscles
Gray text indicates stabilizing muscles
* indicates deep muscles

KNEELING SIDE KICK II

ADVANCED

Alignment and balance are the keys to performing a successful Kneeling Side Kick. Try to articulate each movement through the legs, keeping the spine and hips stable as you kick and flex.

BEST FOR

- gluteus medius
- gluteus maximus
- adductor longus
- rectus abdominis
- transversus abdominis
- pectineus
- adductor longus
- gracilis
- tensor fasciae latae
- sartorius
- rectus femoris
- iliacus
- iliopsoas
- vastus lateralis

DO IT RIGHT

LOOK FOR

- Pressing your weight into your palm on the floor to help maintain balance.
- Keeping your neck long and relaxed.
- Aligning your body so that the shoulders, hips, and legs line up to better activate deep muscles.

AVOID

- Wobbling with movement of the leg—instead, make the movement smaller.

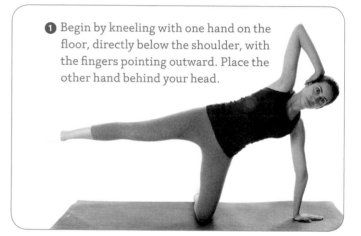

❶ Begin by kneeling with one hand on the floor, directly below the shoulder, with the fingers pointing outward. Place the other hand behind your head.

❷ Lift your top leg to the height of your hip and straighten it, reaching out of your heel. Keep your whole body aligned in one plane so that there is no rotation.

❸ Inhale, and kick your top leg straight out in front of you, flexing your foot and trying not to move at your waist.

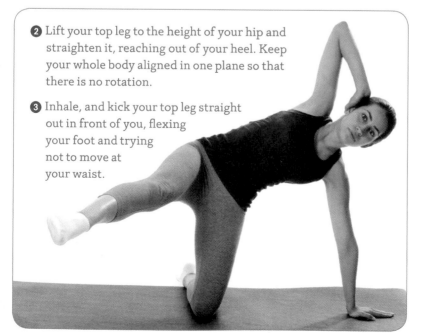

QUICK GUIDE

TARGET

- Leg abductors
- Abdominal muscles

NOT ADVISABLE IF YOU HAVE

- Wrist issues
- Severe back pain
- Shoulder issues
- Pain from lifting above shoulder height

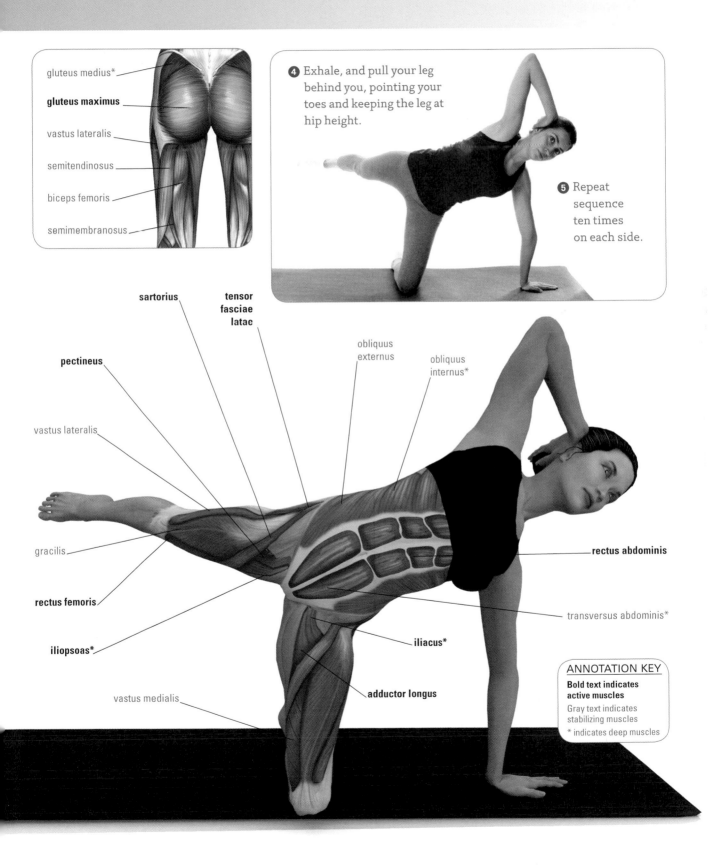

gluteus medius*

gluteus maximus

vastus lateralis

semitendinosus

biceps femoris

semimembranosus

4 Exhale, and pull your leg behind you, pointing your toes and keeping the leg at hip height.

5 Repeat sequence ten times on each side.

sartorius

tensor fasciae latac

pectineus

obliquus externus

obliquus internus*

vastus lateralis

gracilis

rectus abdominis

rectus femoris

transversus abdominis*

iliopsoas*

iliacus*

vastus medialis

adductor longus

ANNOTATION KEY

Bold text indicates active muscles

Gray text indicates stabilizing muscles

* indicates deep muscles

CONTROL BALANCE

Another comprehensive exercise for major lower-body muscles, several fundamental Pilates principles are exemplified in the Control Balance exercise. As in many other exercises, you should distribute your weight evenly, in order to avoid pressure on the neck and spine.

BEST FOR

- gluteus maximus
- gluteus medius
- transversus abdominis
- rectus abdominis
- obliquus externus
- obliquus internus
- tensor fasciae latae
- rectus femoris
- iliacus
- iliopsoas
- vastus lateralis
- vastus medialis
- rectus femoris
- sartorius

ANNOTATION KEY
Bold text indicates active muscles
Gray text indicates stabilizing muscles
* indicates deep muscles

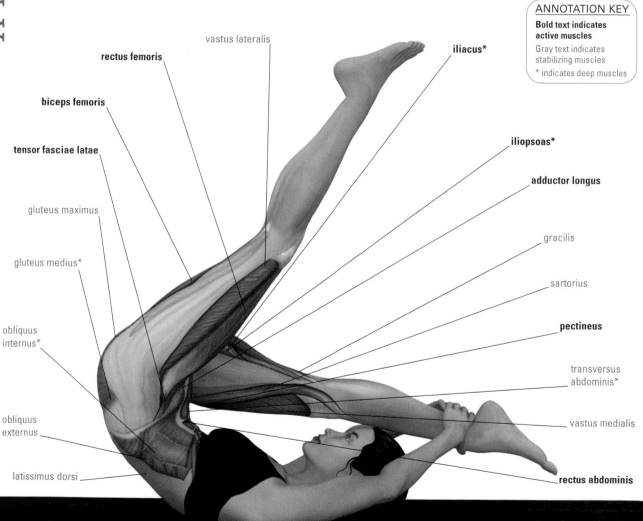

vastus lateralis

rectus femoris

biceps femoris

tensor fasciae latae

gluteus maximus

gluteus medius*

obliquus internus*

obliquus externus

latissimus dorsi

iliacus*

iliopsoas*

adductor longus

gracilis

sartorius

pectineus

transversus abdominis*

vastus medialis

rectus abdominis

① Lie flat on your back with your arms down by your sides, palms facing down and legs in Pilates first position.

② Inhale to prepare. Exhale, and draw your legs up into the air with your inner thighs squeezed and heels together. Inhale, and hold the position.

③ Exhale, press your arms onto the floor, and come to a shoulder stand, lifting your hips and reaching the legs upward.

④ Squeeze your buttocks and draw your navel to your spine to help maintain the hip lift.

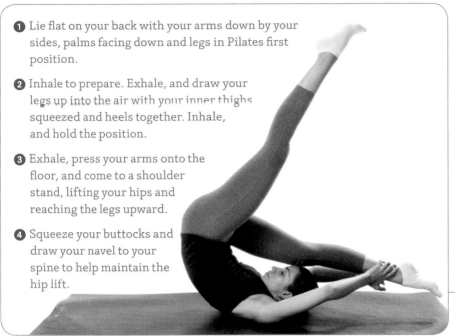

QUICK GUIDE

TARGET
- Gluteal muscles
- Abdominal muscles
- Thigh muscles

BENEFITS
- Builds control and balance

NOT ADVISABLE IF YOU HAVE
- Cervical issues

⑤ Inhale, and lower one leg down toward your head.

⑥ Grab onto your calf with both hands and, at the same time, raise your other leg even higher into the air.

⑦ Pull the calf down for a double-pulse exhale.

⑧ Switch legs and pulse twice.

⑨ Repeat sequence six times on each leg.

DO IT RIGHT

LOOK FOR
- Keeping your hips lifted throughout the exercise.
- Keeping your shoulders drawn down, away from your ears.

AVOID
- Putting weight on your neck—if it is difficult to swallow, there is too much pressure.

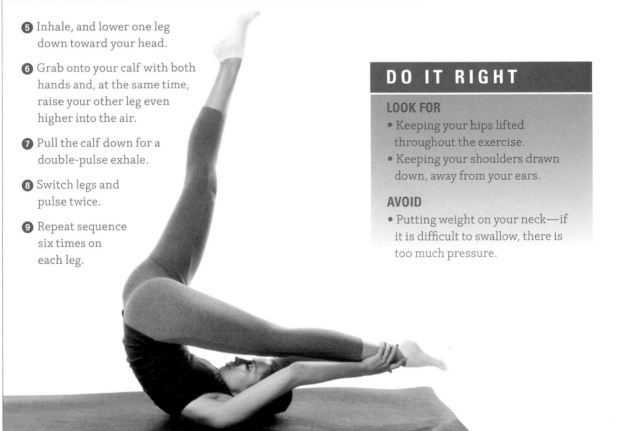

THE STAR

ADVANCED

Performing the ambitious Star exercise targets the upper and lower body, and demonstrates a mastery of Pilates techniques. Allow space for the muscles in all the limbs to lengthen, and maintain balance by eliminating movement in the shoulders and the rest of the body.

BEST FOR

- transversus abdominis
- rectus abdominis
- obliquus internus
- obliquus externus
- vastus lateralis
- vastus medialis
- rectus femoris
- sartorius
- triceps brachii
- deltoideus

QUICK GUIDE

TARGET
- Abdominal muscles
- Thigh muscles

BENEFITS
- Strengthens upper body

NOT ADVISABLE IF YOU HAVE
- Wrist issues
- Neck pain

1 Sit on the side of your hip and prop yourself up on a straight arm, with fingers facing away from your body.

2 Bend your knees and keep your ankles close together, placing your top foot in front (you should be sitting in the Mermaid position).

3 Inhale, press the supporting arm into the floor, and come up into your side plank.

4 Straighten your legs and lift up your hips, reaching your free arm to the sky, keeping the lower arm strong and stable.

5 Exhale, and press the edge of your bottom foot onto the floor as you raise the top leg above the level of your hip.

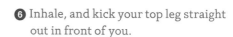

6 Inhale, and kick your top leg straight out in front of you.

7 Flex your foot and try to touch your toes by reaching forward with your top arm, without bending at the waist.

8 Exhale, and kick your leg behind you, pointing your foot.

9 Squeeze your buttocks and keep from arching your back as your top arm reaches for the sky. Repeat sequence three to four times on each side.

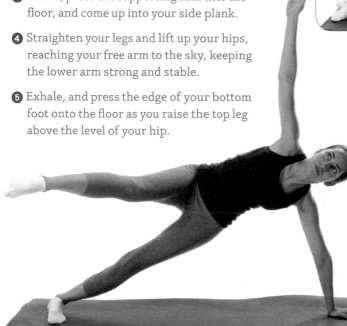

DO IT RIGHT

LOOK FOR
- Lifting your hips up high to take the weight off of your upper body.
- Maintaining stable shoulders by pressing out of the arm and into the floor.
- Trying to keep body movement to a minimum with movement of the arm and leg.
- Pressing through the fingers if the wrist is starting to hurt from pressure.

AVOID
- Allowing your body weight to sink into your wrist and shoulder.
- Pitching forward as you go. Keep your arm directly alongside your ear as you stretch forward.

ANNOTATION KEY
Bold text indicates active muscles
Gray text indicates stabilizing muscles
* indicates deep muscles

gluteus medius*

gluteus maximus

vastus lateralis

semitendinosus

biceps femoris

semimembranosus

teres major

serratus anterior

triceps brachii

obliquus internus*

obliquus externus

brachioradialis

brachialis

rectus abdominis

sartorius

vastus lateralis

rectus femoris

deltoideus

vastus medialis

adductor longus

iliopsoas*

biceps brachii

gracilis

iliacus*

transversus abdominis*

SAMPLE SEQUENCES

ADVANCED

These two sequences of exercises incorporate all of the basics from the Beginner section and the techniques learned in the Intermediate section into an advanced workout series. The Advanced sequences should be performed only after you have mastered the first two sections to ensure safety, precision, and flow. The selected sequences provide a great workout that challenges you to master all of the six principles of Pilates listed in the beginning of this book. These two routines demand that you control your core, and they test your ability to target the proper muscles

MASTERING OF THE CORE I

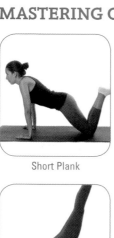
Short Plank

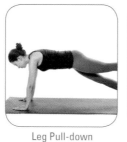
Leg Pull-down

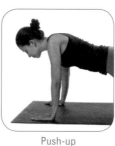
Push-up

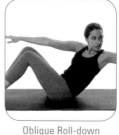
Oblique Roll-down

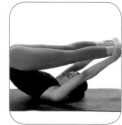
Open-leg Rocker

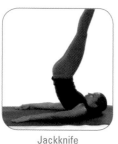
Jackknife

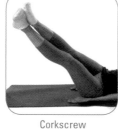
Corkscrew

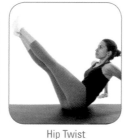
Hip Twist

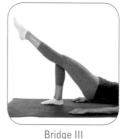
Bridge III

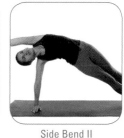
Side Bend II

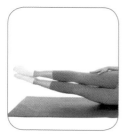
Side Leg Lift

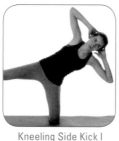
Kneeling Side Kick I

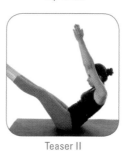
Teaser II

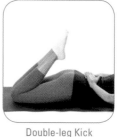
Double-leg Kick

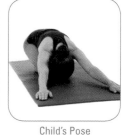
Child's Pose

STRETCHES

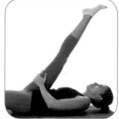
Seal with Foot Clap

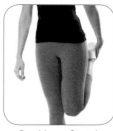
Piriformis Stretch

Hamstring Stretch

Quadriceps Stretch

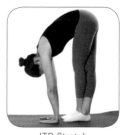
ITB Stretch

and move dynamically using these specific muscles through the entire movement. These exercise sequences are considered advanced because a great deal of control and precision are required to perform them properly. If you are experiencing any difficulty or discomfort with either of these sequences, take time to warm up with some of the Intermediate exercises before attempting an Advanced sequence. Performing the stretches at the end of your workout routine will not only allow your body to cool down, but it will also lengthen and stretch key muscle groups.

MASTERING OF THE CORE II

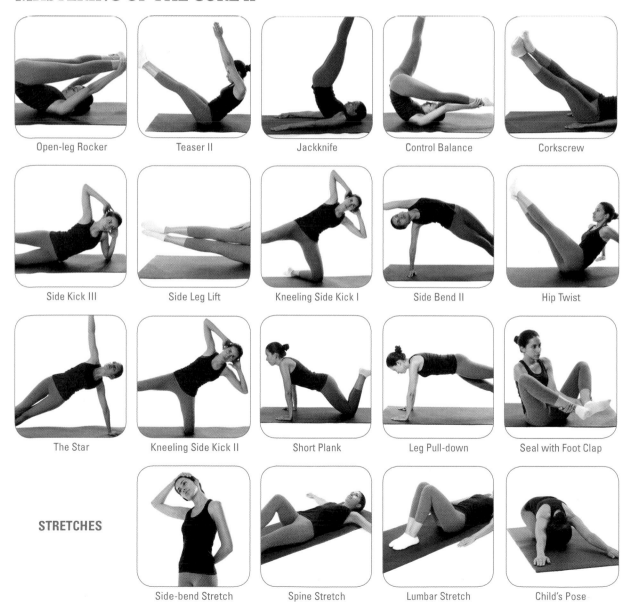

Open-leg Rocker

Teaser II

Jackknife

Control Balance

Corkscrew

Side Kick III

Side Leg Lift

Kneeling Side Kick I

Side Bend II

Hip Twist

The Star

Kneeling Side Kick II

Short Plank

Leg Pull-down

Seal with Foot Clap

STRETCHES

Side-bend Stretch

Spine Stretch

Lumbar Stretch

Child's Pose

CREDITS & ACKNOWLEDGMENTS

All photographs by Jonathan Conklin/Jonathan Conklin Photography

Poster illustrations by Linda Bucklin/Shutterstock

Model: Monica Ordonez

All illustrations by Hector Aiza/3D Labz Animation India, except the insets on pages 18, 20, 22, 23, 24, 25, 26, 29, 30, 41, 47, 61, 70, 79, 93, 99, 101, 105, 109, 112, 115, 121, 129, 131, 133, 135, 137, 139, 143, 147, 149, 151, 153, 157 by Linda Bucklin/Shutterstock

ACKNOWLEDGMENTS

I would like to thank all who helped me prepare this book: To my husband, Tom, for being patient on the weekends, and my clients who diligently proofed the exercises with me. Their hard work and dedication made this book a pleasure to create. I hope you enjoy this book as much as I did putting the material together.

The author and publisher also offer thanks to those closely involved in the creation of this book: Moseley Road president Sean Moore; editor/designer Amy Pierce; art director Brian MacMullen; editorial director/designer Lisa Purcell; and assistant editor Jon Derengowski.